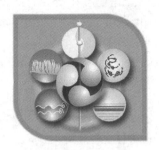

Ayurveda and Acupuncture
Theory and Practice of Ayurvedic Acupuncture
-Marmapuncture (*Siravedhana*)

Dr. Frank Ros

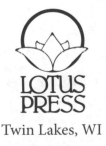

LOTUS PRESS
Twin Lakes, WI

(Co-publication with Waratah Press (Australia) waratahpress@gmail.com)

First Edition, 2014.

Printed in the United States of America

Ros, Frank
Ayurveda and Acupuncture –*Theory and Practice of Ayurvedic Acupuncture*

ISBN:978-0-9406-7624-4

Library of Congress Control Number: 2014945867

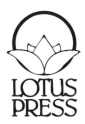

LOTUS PRESS

Published by:
Lotus Press, P.O. Box 325, Twin Lakes, Wisconsin 53181 USA
Web: www.LotusPress.com
e-mail: lotuspress@lotuspress.com
800-824-6396

Table of Contents

Acknowledgement

With much gratitude to:

Professor Dr. P.H. Kulkarni (Ex Ayurvedic Dean, Pune University, India) my research guide and mentor for many years.

The late Professor Dr. Anton Jayasuriya (1930-2005) of Sri Lanka for his great help in the development of Marmapuncture.

Professor Emeritus Dr. Subhash Ranade of Pune, India my current mentor. This book is dedicated to his continuous and untiring work in the international promotion of Ayurveda.

Dr. Carlos Chesta MD of Argentina for his friendship and help in the preparation of the manuscript.

Introductory note from the author

The intention of this book is twofold. On the one hand it is a comprehensive introduction for the layperson to truly understand not only Ayurvedic acupuncture but Ayurveda also.

On the other hand, it is also an in-depth instructional manual for practitioners who practice acupuncture or Ayurveda but would like to learn how to mesh these two together to form an effective, integrative, synergistic system.

I am heartened to learn the interest around the world on this little known system of acupuncture since my first book in 1994, I have received many emails from readers and which have resulted in me visiting the US a number of times and South America to lecture on the subject. A postgraduate course for Ayurvedic practitioners in Perth, Australia, has been an inspiring guiding light for me to continue with this work. The support I have received from a number of Indian experts such as Professors Ranade and Lele besides others is exemplary.

It is amazing what one can achieve with a simple tool like a filiform needle and some substantial knowledge handed down from the ancient rishis but which can be utilized today to a great effect.

It is also humbling to accept that because of the incredible international promotion of acupuncture by my Chinese colleagues, that the interest in acupuncture in general has facilitated a quicker acceptance internationally of Ayurvedic acupuncture in particular.

I hope the following work inspires the reader into further research. Ayurveda is a great, open natural science and its philosophy and methods are as applicable today as they once were thousands of years ago. It gives us the understanding via a holistic perspective, possibly one of the most holistic systems in the world.

Dr. Frank Ros
Australia
May, 2013

Prologue

The International Academy of Ayurveda (IAA) is the premier institution in India for the international teaching and promotion of Ayurveda and for international students of Ayurveda. We work closely with our local universities in India in order to maintain an excellent standard of Ayurvedic teaching worldwide. Our professional staff has taught in many countries including Europe, Canada, USA, Brazil, Argentina, Chile, Australia, Russia, China and Japan.

Marma therapy and Ayurvedic acupuncture or Siravedhana, (also commonly called Marmapuncture) is a specialized field stemming from ancient Shalya Chikitsa and originally taught as a therapy by the Dhanvantari surgical school in ancient India. Although originally banned in India by the colonial powers along with Ayurveda, Ayurvedic acupuncture is once again slowly beginning to be practiced in India and Sri Lanka.

We are pleased to acknowledge our strong connection with Dr. Frank Ros, a colleague and facilitator of Ayurvedic acupuncture teaching.

Frank, besides being the author of an authoritative book on Ayurvedic acupuncture (1994) is also the author of a chapter in one of our recent internationally-released books *Ayurveda and Marma Therapy* (Lotus Press. USA)- written by Dr. S. Ranade, Dr. A. Lele and Dr. D. Frawley.

He has taught in Australia and overseas for a number of years. We have found Frank to be a knowledgeable and skilled practitioner and lecturer and we highly recommend him.

The IAA currently provides certification for international postgraduate students of Ayurveda, who major in Ayurvedic acupuncture as specifically taught by Dr. Ros.

Prof. Em. Dr. Subhash Ranade Chairman,
International Academy of Ayurveda
Pune
(ex-Ayurvedic Dean, Pune University)
(ex-Principal of Ashtanga Ayurveda College, Pune, India)

Prof. Dr. Avinash Lele
Vice-Chairman, *International Academy of Ayurveda*
Pune
Professor, Department of Shalya Chikitsa
(Post Graduate section) *Tilak Ayurved Mahavidyalaya College.*
Pune, Maharashtra, India.

Introduction

During the course of time there has been a constant effort by all people in the pursuit of happiness. In different cultures and at different times there have developed a wide range of methods both physical and existential to overcome pain.

Although many of these methods appear to be very different, actually all reflect the need to overcome human suffering. It is within this same context that is the theme or point of this book, to provide people with useful information on the ancient science of acupuncture, approached from the perspective of traditional Indian medicine known as Ayurveda. Interestingly, the term for needle in Chinese is bian which means stone and demonstrates just how ancient acupuncture really is.

Ayurveda is an ancient science developed over thousands of years in India by sages called rishis, who left this legacy of wisdom and knowledge for the benefit of mankind. The knowledge of acupuncture points on the body surface which may be used for therapeutic purposes have been developed both within Ayurveda and in traditional Chinese medicine. The latter, in particular, undoubtedly the most widespread acupuncture system today has become a very important method of treating diseases.

Ayurveda is a living science that adapts to living beings and their needs. For a very long time, the knowledge of the points have been known in Ayurveda as siras and marmas but was quite relegated to certain circles, people, in general, within families-that transmitted this knowledge without revealing it publicly.

For this reason, among others, Ayurvedic acupuncture, known as suchi-karma, had no development in modern times as important as Chinese acupuncture, although this knowledge was always there in the main texts of Ayurveda. In fact, recent research conducted by doctors B. K. Joshi, R. L. Shah and G. Joshi demonstrate that the knowledge of the points (siras), meridians (dhamanis) and vital areas (marmas) was duly mentioned in the Sushruta Samhita, a classic text of Ayurveda, written several thousands years ago (500 B.C.). However, these terms were misinterpreted henceforth with the passage of time and wrongly translated as simply veins, arteries and places that were not to be injured during surgery, and that the marmas concept is based purely on their susceptibility to injury or death. However, it's rewarding to learn that these points or areas may also be used to treat various health problems.

With the passage of time and the decrease of cultural differences, these concepts that were dormant and largely hidden, often because they were banned by the colonial powers that controlled India for a long time are beginning to be revealed once again for the benefit of all people, irrespective of race, culture or religion.

The Ayurvedic acupuncture system integrates the concept of meridians and points [known as dhamanis and siras] and also uses its internationally-accepted numbering system (nomenclature) similar to Chinese acupuncture, while also incorporating the benefits of the wisdom of Ayurveda. The unwary reader may mistakenly think that this book is a synthesis of the concepts of traditional medicines of India and China. However, actually this is an important step for the integration between these two sciences which, although appearing different, in fact share the same basic principles, energy, movement, the concept of nature, the five elements, etc. – since as much of their knowledge have the same historical roots. Therefore, the principles and techniques of Ayurveda can be used in perfect harmony by practitioners of most schools of acupuncture.

However, we must not forget that any kind of knowledge or technique used in medicine can be useless if it has no practical application, and it is just then, when people have the opportunity to practice suchi-karma that it may reveal its effectiveness.

Sometimes one can fall in the trap of discussing whether this technique or that technique corresponds to a particular place or who owns the knowledge, but it loses its meaning when one comes face to face with suffering, and it is at this point that the real answer lies when these methods serve to mitigate the pain and suffering of people all over the world.

Although this knowledge has been kept secret for a long time, as a way to keep alive this teaching, in these new times predominated by communication, it is a must to disclose and make public its use as part of our heritage as human beings. These techniques should be employed to maintain the integrity of peoples' health in both its physical and spiritual aspects, and not to manipulate or generate more imbalances, because in that way we once again justify its concealment as it occurred before, which is not appropriate for these modern times.

It is a moral obligation to integrate and unify all health knowledge so they can be accessed in a simple and clear way by everyone. Just think about all the diseases and problems that can be avoided by utilizing the knowledge of acupuncture and complementary medicines within the field of traditional medical practice.

Therefore, I hope this book will be useful for those interested in the science of healing. It is my sincere hope that those who come across suchi karma will find it very useful and a source of personal satisfaction, as it has been for me, and to those skilled in natural medicine, that it may serve as an incentive to remain on track to improve the health of the world.

I am most happy to have been able to collaborate with my colleague Dr. Frank Ros in the publication of this book *Ayurveda And Acupuncture*.

Dr. Carlos D. Chesta, MD
March 2013
Rosario, Argentina
Dr. Chesta is a medical doctor and professor of Ayurveda at the National University of Rosario, Argentina and uses marmapuncture in his clinic.

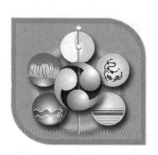

History and principles of ayurveda

Ayurveda

In Sanskrit, Ayurveda means Ayus- life, longevity and Veda- means knowledge, wisdom or science, thus the term The Science of Life. It is also described as the Indian science for maintaining life, which includes not only therapeutics but also preventive treatments and lifestyle.

History

The history of Ayurveda extends back to time immemorial but is generally described in the Vedas, regarded as probably the oldest written documentation of life and medicine in the world.

The Vedas are sacred writings much in the form of poems or chants and describing a variety of knowledge which was considered essential for health of body, mind and spirit.

Ayurveda is a subsidiary Veda (Upaveda), but in many aspects it is considered the uppermost Veda.

Vedas

There are four major written classics or Vedas which were originally carefully memorized and passed on from parent to child for countless generations prior to the information being written down. These four are:

• Rig Veda

Basic foundation of the other Vedas and oldest, consisting of ten texts or books (10,572 verses).

• Yajur Veda

40 chapters of verses

• Sama Veda

Repetition of Rig Veda plus additional verses and material

• Atharva Veda

Recognized as the most comprehensive of the four Vedas, with regards to Ayurvedic Medicine.

Ayurveda is considered as having developed from the Rig Veda, It is thought that the knowledge was received or perceived by the Rishis or great ancient seers of wisdom, some experts explain this occurred during meditative states of the Rishis near the Himalayas or great mountains of Northern India. The seers were almost always expert doctors and their methods were highly regarded by the governments and peoples of India.

An additional Veda written several thousand years later (1000 BC) is the Suchi Veda which is a comprehensive compilation of needling (acupuncture) techniques. However, there are other techniques of needling (e.g. suturing) mentioned also and demonstrates the irrefutable connection in ancient India between surgery and acupuncture. The Suchi Veda is delegated as an Upaveda or subsidiary minor writing of the Vedas. Perhaps it should have been titled Suchi Samhita instead.

Dhanvantari is regarded as the most ancient, greatest seer of Ayurveda. He lived in Benares, India.

Eight Branches

Later (about 1000 BC) the medical principles described in the Vedas were scientifically systemized, collated and expand upon, they were also put through various rigorous tests to prove their efficacy. This resulted in the formation of eight distinct branches of Ayurveda (Ashtanga Ayurveda) which included pediatrics, surgery, toxicology, internal medicine, psychiatry, rejuvenation and so forth.

Also, there occurred the establishment of two distinct schools of Ayurveda, the Atreya School of physicians and the Dhanvantari School of surgeons.

Concurrently, various other written compilations following in the footsteps of the Vedas were written, of which only three remain today, the others becoming extinct. These three (samhitas) are referred to as the Great Trio.

Samhitas

These three compilations described the concepts of Ayurveda for posterity, which were only previously available in writing within the four Vedas.

The Charaka Samhita is attributed to the great physician Charaka and is a monumental treatise on the general concepts of Ayurveda, including herbal and other allied therapies.

The Sushruta Samhita is attributed to the great ancient Indian surgeon Sushruta and is similarly a monumental work on surgery. Some of its surgical concepts are being today evaluated and proving to be in some cases more effective than the modern surgical techniques. Even acupuncture was mentioned by Sushruta and was taught at the Dhanvantari School in ancient India according to Prof. Dr. H.S. Sharma, former Ayurvedic Dean at Gujarat University.[1]

The Ashtanga Hridaya Samhita is attributed to Vagbhatta and itself is a synthesis of both the Charaka and Sushruta Samhitas. Vagbhatta was a Buddhist who revitalized Ayurveda by his writings and it was Buddhism in its heydays that greatly and successfully promoted Ayurveda within India and abroad, to the East.

Ancient History

Ayurveda has been suppressed or even banned by a number of different invaders of India, but most noticeably, the British colonizers. They removed all traces of this science to supplant it with western medical training and practice, so as to produce a ready market for their medicines and drugs. The British were allegedly very big in 'Westernizing' the Orientals. Very traditional practitioners continued to practice Ayurveda under fear of being caught and teaching was necessarily done by word of mouth, in secret.

Much earlier than this, according to scholars the Muslim conquerors attempted to destroy matters dealing with what they termed 'pagan religion' and in so doing destroyed many valuable works on Ayurveda, acupuncture and many other systems (1000-1200 AD). For instance, Nalanda University (400- 1200 AD) was reputed to have had an international standing and had 10,000 students, 1500 teachers and numerous other staff. Tens of thousands of literary works

1 Dr.H.S.Sharma (ExDean of Gujarat University) from Vedic Health Care System by Drs. B.K.Joshi, R.L.Shah, G.Joshi. New Age Books New Delhi. 2002. (FOREWORD).

were reportedly destroyed with only some escaping the onslaught and ending up in Tibet. In fact, some ancient Ayurvedic texts are only today available in the Tibetan language. Nalanda University taught a very wide range of subjects including astrology, medicine and acupuncture, but it was totally destroyed.

Prior to this period, Alexander the Great (c. 356-323 BC), the great Macedonian king, after invading the greater part of India accepted the Ayurvedic physicians' great ability in healing and officially took back with him a number of Ayurvedists to try expand Greek medicine. It is alleged that Alexander was so impressed by the Ayurvedic physicians that he ordered all his troops only be treated by the Ayurvedic practitioners and methods.

Emperor Ashoka (c. 304–232 BC) was converted to Buddhism and in so doing promoted Ayurveda to an incredible extent, not only throughout India but into neighboring countries also.

Universities, hospitals and other medical institutions were set up to train practitioners and to treat the population. A three-tier system of physicians was established (a) royal physicians (b) private physicians for private patients and (c) public physicians (free to the public).

Sri Lanka, about this time received Ayurvedic medicine and acupuncture within Buddhism which it embraced wholeheartedly. It is recorded that Emperor Ashoka's son, Mahinda, himself a Buddhist monk was the first to introduce the system to Sri Lanka.

Modern India
After Mahatma Ghandi's attempt to free India and the end of colonial domain, India has once again embarked on promoting Ayurveda. 1972 saw the acceptance by the government of the Ayurvedic Pharmacopoeia. 1995 has seen the acceptance of Ayurveda as an equal to orthodox medicine, with government funding distributed equally to Ayurvedic universities, medical colleges and hospitals along with its conventional counterpart. Today, the future of Ayurvedic medicine and acupuncture (Suchi Karma) looks excellent not only within India, but also internationally.

What exactly is Ayurveda?

Introduction to Ayurveda
Ayurveda is the traditional medical system of India, practiced for more than seven thousand years.

Ayurveda is based on many therapeutic methods that share the same principles or philosophy of natural medicine based on the Vedic system. The diagnosis and treatment follow the same path in order to establish balance in the human body.

Tridosha

The science of Ayurveda is distinct from other forms of medicine simply by the Tridosha theory. This theory explains about three subtle forces that exist in the body and directing all body functions.

These three energies are called Vata (which has a connection to the wind or air) Pitta (which connects to heat) and Kapha (related to the cold, congestion and muscle growth, weight gain etc.). Everyone has these three energies but in different amounts or percentages. For example, a person can have a seventy percent of Pitta, a ten percent of Vata and twenty percent of Kapha. Thus, the person may feel more the heat than the cold and for that reason may prefer the cold rather than heat.

Tridosha is the science of the three humoral energies. These three are the driving forces behind all body functions. They are the center or heart of Ayurveda. The Tridosha is a term of generalization of the energies of Vata, Pitta and Kapha (VPK) all of which derive from Prana or biological energy (the Chinese call it Ch'i). Tri translates as 'three' and dosha as 'fault', called fault because when they are adversely affected by an imbalance, then they can also generate a failure, a disease. Its quality is negatively reflected in the body, e.g. dry skin and nervous tension for Vata.

Vata

The subtle energy called Vata directs all movements, whether of nerves, hormones, muscles etc. Also causes catabolism in the body.

Pitta

The subtle energy called Pitta leads to digestion and metabolism.

Kapha

The subtle energy called Kapha leads to anabolism or body growth.

Tridoshas body sites

In Ayurveda it is believed that the humor / Kapha dosha originates in the stomach, its principal or primary organ and from here its energy ascends or descends depending on the time of day. When it exceeds its limit, it moves to other parts of the body and causes harm, for example the lung where it causes congestion.

Similarly, Pitta originates in the small intestine, which is its principal or primary organ. When aggravated after exceeding its limit, it moves to other parts of the body and causes harm, for example inflammation of joints. The liver is the secondary organ of Pitta.

Vata originates in the large intestine, which is the main organ or primary site of Vata. When aggravated after exceeding its limit, it is transmitted to other parts of the body to cause harm, for example dry skin. The kidney is the secondary organ of Vata, which dries out the body by removing water. This primary and secondary sites concept of the doshas and the organs is important as will be seen later in the text.

Pancha Karma treatment is to remove the excess dosha, which builds out from its parent organ, causing damage (e.g. knee) and returns it to its parent organ, then from there to remove the excess dosha. Once the dosha is back to its proper level, health is restored.

In the body, there are three areas that are affected by the Tridoshas. Kapha, under the control of the stomach, affects the torso about from the neck to the diaphragm. Pitta, under the control of the small intestine, affects the torso approximately from the diaphragm to the umbilicus. Vata, under the control of the Large Intestine affects the torso approximately from the umbilicus to the groin (and also affects the legs). The proper balance of these three areas also called Tridosha, has its own pranic channel (dhamani) called the Tridosha dhamani, which controls and balances these three doshic areas. These reflections of the doshas on other parts of the body will be discussed later in the text.

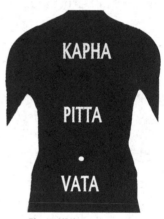

Fig. 1. VPK sites

The Five Elements

However, Tridosha is not the only concept of Ayurveda. Since ancient times, Ayurveda has also taught the concept of the Five Elements (*Pancha Maha-Bhutas - Five Great Elements*). These five elements form the substrate of Ayurveda and are closely connected with the Tridosha. The five elements are critical in acupuncture.

The ancient teacher Charaka says that the universe is developed from these five from subtle to physical, it is argued that before them there is Prana or vital energy, this energy is attached to the *ether*, space and develops wind or air (*Vayu*), followed by Fire (*Agni*), Water (*Ap*) and finally *Earth* (*Prithvi*), the most physical of the five. All things are composed of these elements, but only living beings also have Prana which directs the body.

It is most interesting to learn that the Chinese medical system did not have this knowledge of the Five Elements and *Tsou Yen* at about 200BC was the person who included it in China after receiving Ayurvedic concepts from the Indians, through Buddhism [2].

> *"The great works (Samhita) which make up the corpus of Ayurvedic medicine, were founded (like the other four sciences of India) on the theories of the breath[Prana], of the humors [Vata Pitta Kapha] and of the constituent [5] elements of the microcosm and macrocosm. This was a very different conception from the Chinese hypothesis, referring only to the two principles (yin-yang) and the eight trigrams [bagua] to account for the perpetual transformation of things, whether in the physical or moral world."* [3]

In Japan, which also received Buddhism and the principles of Ayurveda, the Five Elements are called *'Godai'* which means the 'Great Five' and follow the same plan of Ayurveda, Ether (space, empty) Wind / Air, Fire , Water and Earth.

In acupuncture, the Five Elements explain the connections between the meridians or *dhamanis*, as well as the qualities of many acupoints or *siras*. The treatment of fire (inflammation) for instance, can be done effectively in both the meridians (dhamanis) that relate directly to fire, in addition to the points or siras with Fire attributes.

Tridosha and the Five Elements

The three doshas are energies while the five elements are substances but both are concepts that go together. It is due to the physical elements that the body has a field in which to act and is due to the doshas (VPK) by which the elements receive prana, life.

The doshas are formed via the Five Elements and Prana. Vata is Ether and Wind, united (by Prana), Pitta is Fire and Water, united (by Prana) and Kapha is Water and Earth united (by Prana). *Prana* gives them life, as a body without prana has the elements but is dead and the vital points, the *marmas* (lethal/ vital zones) disappear when there is no prana in the body.

> *"Marmas exists only when prana is present in the body, a dead body does not have any marma and it's fully activated only when prana actually moves through the marma."* [4]

The qualities of the five elements and the doshas are recognized in people by their constitution *or Prakruti*.

2 Prof. P. Huard and Dr. M. Wong. Chinese Medicine. World University Press, London. UK. (p.12).
3 Ibid. (p.88).
4 Svoboda R., *Ayurveda, Life, Health and Vitality,* Penguin Publishers USA 1993. (p.65).

Constitution	Element	Quality
Vata-	Ether and Wind,	dry, mobile, cold, catabolism
Pitta-	Fire and Water,	hot, wet, metabolism
Kapha-	Water and Earth,	cold, motionless, anabolism

Prakruti

The *Prakruti* (constitution) of each person can also be recognized by the qualities that manifest in the person. Although we have the three doshas, one is normally a dominant dosha.

Vata Person

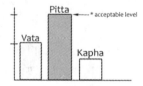

Pitta Person

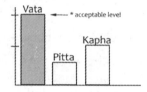

Kapha Person

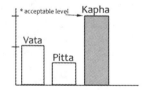

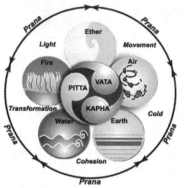

Fig 2. The 5 Elements and 3 Doshas

Qualities of the constitution (Prakruti)

Vata

Vata types are tall or short in stature, have thin, dry and cold skin, visible veins, small head, small eyes, nose and thin lips, small hands and feet, variable appetite, emotionally responds with fear, nervousness and anxiety. They have a rapid pulse with quality of a *snake* in its erratic, slithery movement.

Pitta
Pitta types have medium height, with moderate muscles, moderate weight, reddish complexion (Fire), hot skin and a small amount of fat, moderate head size, but may have mild eye inflammation, medium nose and lips, medium hands and feet and hot, strong appetite and emotionally respond with anger or irritability. They have a moderate, even pulse with a shape not unlike a hopping frog (*poing, poing, poing!*)

Kapha
Kapha types have small stature but are strong, may have a pale complexion (water), cold, wet and white skin, large head size, wide eyes, prominent nose and thick lips, big and cold hands and feet, poor but constant appetite, responds emotionally by calm, are sentimental and happy. They have a deep, slow and relaxed pulse with a smooth movement like a *swan.*

Therapies
In Ayurveda there are several forms of ancient therapies such as massage, applying heat to the marmas or vital areas (acupoints) called *agni-karma*, application of special oils, as well as a special treatment called *Pancha Karma* itself consisting of five therapies. *Pancha Karma* (Five Therapies) is used to remove toxins, return the Tridoshas (VPK) back to their acceptable positions in the body and thus maintain health.

When there is a disease, the dosha or fault (either excess Vata, Pitta or Kapha) is transferred to places such as the knee where it can cause damage (e.g. arthritis). Pancha Karma helps return this dosha back to its place of origin and into a state of equilibrium.

Therapies also used are precious stones and colors, meditation, yoga and diet.

Herbology
Herbs are also used as medicine but in Ayurveda it is necessary to know the most important qualities before ingesting. For example, the effect of an increase or decrease of the energy of an herb it will have based on the qualities of Tridosha and the Five Elements.

When a person with mostly Vata e.g., consumes an herb that increases Vata (V+) then this can result in an imbalance and in the end causes an imbalance of Vata dosha type. Its proper treatment in this case is to consume an herb that reduces Vata (V-) by its qualities. As Vata has two qualities, dry and cold, then the therapy more acceptable to reduce the excessive level of Vata (V+) is a therapy / or herb or a combination, with qualities of heat and moisture to reduce the Vata that is in excess.

Meals and beverages have a similar effect on the doshas and therefore when a person consumes a meal that increases Vata, the person with Vata constitution may be negatively affected, especially if that food or drink is consumed often. Ayurveda advises appropriate diets for each type of person. These qualities are called Guna dvandva qualities of opposition. For example, the effect of the dry Vata (air) can reduce or treat the wet or oily quality of Kapha (Water). Pitta, the heating effect can be reduced by the cold of Kapha. Moisture and coldness of Kapha can be remedied by the heat of Pitta (Fire).

In Ayurveda, a combination of herbal teas for Vata constitution person (Vatik) can not contain herbs to dry and give cold, as these increase Vata possibly beyond the level acceptable to that person and thus place their health at risk. The correct treatment would be to use a combination of plants yielding heat but which do not dry the body.

For example, useful for Vata type are the use of garlic, ajwan, cinnamon, ashwagandha, ginger, nutmeg, cardamom, valerian, etc.

Guna dvandva

Guna dvandva means qualities of the opposites. Treatment of one may be carried out by the use of its opposite, for example, cold is treated by heat. It is somewhat akin to the principles of yin-yang.

The Opposite Qualities

Heavy (*guru*)	Light (*laghu*)
Cold (*sita*)	Hot (*ushna*)
Wet or greasy (*snigdha*)	Dry (*ruksa*)
Slow (*send*)	Fast (*tiksna*)
Static (*sthira*)	Mobile (*sara*)
Soft (*urdu*)	Hard (*kathina*)
Clear (*vishada*)	Turbid (*picchila*)

Tastes

In Ayurveda the tastes are considered very important because they may increase or decrease the Five Elements and the Tridoshas (VPK). The tastes can cure while those which are wrong for the patient can do harm. Ayurveda recognizes six flavors or tastes. They are used as a guide to proper diet from food according to the doshas.

Taste	Effect	Elements
Sweet	Cold	Earth and Water
Salty	Heat	Fire and Water
Sour	Heat	Earth and Fire
Bitter	Cold	Air and Ether
Pungent	Heat	Fire and Air
Astringent	Cold	Air and Earth

The sweet taste, such as sugar can increase Kapha and cause weight gain because it is formed of Water and Earth. The Salty taste (e.g. salt) can increase Pitta and cause inflammation, as can heat (e.g. pepper, Fire and Air). Bitter taste (lemon) can increase Vata by its elements of Air and Ether and also with Astringent (pomegranate), for its constituent of Air. The Pungent taste can be tolerated by Vata due to its element of Fire, but if consumed in quantity, can aggravate Vata by its element of Air.

Diagnosis
Ayurveda uses various forms of diagnoses. One such important consideration is the radial pulse.

Pulse
The pulse shows several features that help the practitioner to determine what actually happens in the body, the cause of the disease and not just the symptoms. The practitioner uses three fingers on the patient's arm near the wrist. The index finger is used to determine the status of Vata (1), the middle finger for Pitta (2) and ring finger for Kapha (3), in the right arm as well as on the left. These three positions also determine the states of the organs. With light touch the state of the hollow organs (e.g. large intestine) are revealed while with a heavier touch, the state of the solid organs (e.g. heart) can be determined.

The quality of the pulse can demonstrate the condition of a certain dosha e.g. a snake/slippery feel on the fingers for Vata.

Left radial pulse	Right radial pulse
(1) *Vata* (snake)	*Vata* (snake)
Heart / Small Intestine	Lung / Large Intestine
(2) *Pitta* (frog)	*Pitta* (frog)
Spleen / Stomach	Liver / Gallbladder
(3) *Kapha* (swan)	*Kapha* (swan)
Kidney / Bladder	Pericardium / Tridoshas

The observation of the lips, face, eyes, nails and tongue are also used for diagnosis.

Tongue

The tongue shows reflections of the body and when it does not work well, it tends to show a stain, dryness etc. in the positions of these organs represented on the tongue.

For example, toxins (*ama*) in the gastro-intestinal tract appear as a white area in the center of the tongue (tongue coating). Kidney problems appear on the sides and near the base of the tongue, while lung problems are at the sides and tip of the tongue. Thus all the organs are represented on the tongue.

Nails

Vata nails are usually fragile and brittle, Pitta's are soft and pink, while Kapha's are thick, heavy and greasy.

Acupuncture

It may be surprising for some to read an inclusion on acupuncture in a book on Ayurveda, but it should come as no surprise since acupuncture itself is a very ancient art, its actual origins are shrouded in mystery.

> *"There is proof that acupuncture has been practiced in ancient Egypt, Persia, India, Sri Lanka, many parts of Europe and South America, and even by the North American Indians."* [5]

One of the earliest written records on acupuncture (if not the earliest) is found in the Vedic writings. Acupuncture was called *Siravedhana* (*siras* or acupoints punctured with a needle) in ancient Ayurveda.

> *"In the three major Ayurvedic texts, discussions of surgery and marma points also involved Ayurvedic acupuncture or "needling", and moxibustion. The use of needles was used for both surgical and non-surgical healing. It was first recorded in the Suchi Veda (science of needling) about 3000 years ago."* [6]

It was used also as part of surgery (Shalya Chikitsa) and the ancient surgeon and teacher Sushruta (500BC) explains in his authoritative book *Sushruta Samhita* that there are 700 siras (acupoints) in the body that are embedded in the 24 *dhamanis* or channels (meridians) of Prana [7]. The practitioner uses fine needles (filiform needles) to carefully puncture the *sira*, so as not to cause discomfort to the patient. This causes a reaction in the sira which is transmitted through

---

5 Dr. John Veltheim. *Acupuncture.* Hill of Content. Melb. Australia. (p.1)
6 Swami Sada Shiva Tirtha. *The Ayurveda Encyclopedia.* Ayurveda Holistic Center Press, NY. USA. (pg 556).
7 Drs. B.K.Joshi, R.L.Shah, G.Joshi. *Vedic Health Care System.* (p.viii).

the body via the prana flowing through the pranic channels (dhamanis and nadis). The reaction may be remote as well as local when puncturing the sira. An organ like the liver can be treated remotely, by piercing the appropriate sira on the skin of the foot or can treat the affected foot by the local sira. Ayurvedic acupuncture uses the same system of Ayurveda, the use of the theory of Tridosha, the Five Elements and the various forms of diagnoses. It's usually used in combination with massage treatments, herbs and Pancha Karma. It is the same system but varies only by needling the points (siras) and areas/zones (Marma) where other practitioners may often use massage.

In India and Sri Lanka today, acupuncture based on Vedic principles is somewhat secretive and protected by traditional practitioners.

"According to Dr. V. Dharmalingam, there exists a small group of Siddha and Ayurvedic practitioners in South India who use gold and copper needles to acupuncture certain vital points. Sri Lanka appears to possess an indigenous form of therapeutic acupuncture. Numerous documents on Sinhalese Buddhist and Ayurvedic medicine written on palm-leaf attest to the ancient use of fine acupuncture needles (22 recorded types).

A study done by Laxman Devasena entitled Some Traditional Sri Lankan Medical Techniques Related to Acupuncture, 'reveals a system of great breadth and long history. In Sri Lanka even today many practitioners use these ancient techniques both on humans and animals."[8]

Chapter 2 describes the history and structure of siravedhana or Vedic acupuncture. The above Ayurvedic principles will be further elucidated and discussed in the chapters to follow.

8 Dr. Robert Svoboda and Arnie Lade. *Tao and Dharma.* Lotus Press, WI. USA (1995) (p.144).

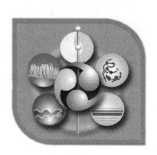

History and philosophy
of ayurvedic acupuncture

Definition

As previously discussed, the word 'Ayurvedic' stems from two Sanskrit words-
Ayus meaning Life and *Veda* meaning Science thus its combined form means
the 'Science of Life'.

The word 'acupuncture' on the other hand is derived from *acus* which is Latin
for needle and *puncture*, so it means 'puncturing with a needle' and it is a long
standing medical technique for lancing or drawing fluids out of tissues by the
use of a surgical needle. It resembles Oriental acupuncture only by the use of
needles. [9]

Ayurvedic acupuncture therefore can be defined as:

'The traditional Indian system of needling strategic pressure points on the body
to cure or prevent disease, according to Ayurvedic principles'.

Traditionally though, Ayurvedic acupuncture has also been called '*Suchi Karma*'
in Sanskrit- the traditional language of India. *Suchi* means a needle, *karma*
means therapy thus it means 'needle therapy'.

---

9 Acupuncture is a term given by Western medical doctors to the needling techniques (Chinese- *zhen*) they observed when visiting China during President Nixon's visit in 1972 as it resembled the Western technique via use of needles.

Explanation about acupuncture

Acupuncture needles (also called *filiform needles*) are inserted at various pressure points of the body (known as *marmas* and *siras*) which like a pearl necklace, are connected together by a common thread or channel (*nadi*). Bio-energy (*Prana*) travels along each channel and then concentrates at each pressure point. A disease is simply an imbalance in this energy and its transmission along the channels, so that by puncturing the points, the energy can be balanced and health re-established.

Each of the twelve major organs of the body (e.g. heart, liver, kidney etc.) are similarly located along this 'necklace' just like the points, so that there is really one long loop (*nadi* or channel), connecting with various points (over 700) which are themselves separated by the organs. In reality, this long thread or *nadi* is itself made up of separate sections often called *dhamanis* (like Pranic arteries).

History

The history of Ayurvedic acupuncture is inter-twined with the history of Ayurveda itself and can be traced back in India to at least 7-9 thousand years ago. Recently, various excavations in India have given extra credibility to the above with regards to the antiquity of Ayurveda.

> *"The rediscovery of the ancient Sarasvati River system and the Mehrgarh site, shows an organic development of civilization in India going back to 6500 BC. with a strong Vedic presence from the earliest era, thus giving much greater antiquity to Vedic culture, of which Ayurveda is a part, than has been previously thought."* [10]

Since very ancient times, humans throughout the world have utilized various methods in order to heal themselves. These consisted of preparing herbs or plants, which were in abundance, into a poultice for treating external injuries or else mixing with food for internal medicine. Later, as other substances were discovered they were added to the known gamut of remedies, finally developing into a comprehensive catalogue (materia medica) of natural substances which could be used as healing adjuncts. Some of these substances were used in everyday food preparation like spices, which later became highly sought-after ingredients; others were mainly used as medicines in the event of a dis-ease or as prevention. Concurrently, massage with the hand of an afflicted part of the body became sensical and thus various masso-therapy techniques were developed.

Due to injuries sustained while either fighting enemy tribes or else from marauding animals, humans began to develop other more physical forms of

---

10 Dr. David Frawley, in *The Lost Secrets of Ayurvedic Acupuncture*, by Dr. Frank Ros, Lotus Publications Wi, U.S.A. 1994. (Foreword).

healing. One of these was obviously the removal of a foreign object (e.g. from the eye) or else a weapon such as an arrow, inflicted during a struggle with the enemy. Here too, various techniques and knowledge were developed by necessity in order for the tribe to survive. This was the forerunner of later surgical techniques.

Readily available objects like timber, animal bones and stones were often fashioned into instruments for fighting the enemy. A wooden club (or small branch of a tree) was ideal for hitting an opponent. Later, timber was fashioned into objects which could puncture the skin of the animal or human and penetrate through to injure or kill. This was the concept of the arrow and spear. Also, stones were fashioned into crude axe blades with a cutting edge and tied to a wooden handle by a thong. A blade was not only used to kill or injure a living being but also could be used to cut and fashion meat and food. Later, knives would develop from this.

Suturing

Large wounds would be found to heal slowly and often open up again. It was soon realized that some form of stitching the two open surfaces together would provide a more stable and quicker healing method. This became the knowledge of suturing where a thread (attached to a needle) is passed through the flesh to 'sew' the wound together. Various plants were discovered to be poisonous and thus to be avoided or else possess special qualities which could daze, put to sleep or numb an area of the body.

For instance, the plant grown in India and called the Indian Snake Plant (*Rauwolfia Serpentina*) was found to produce a tranquillizing effect which could be used to put someone in a deep sleep and unaware of pain while suturing etc.

"The golden age of Ayurvedic medicine coincides with Buddhism's period of ephemeral glory in India (327BC-750 AD) and the great period of continental and maritime expansion which carried India's influence abroad. Among the Buddha's attendants there featured two doctors, Kasparja and Jivaka, the last of whom later became a patron of Tibetan medicine to whom tradition ascribes extraordinary operations carried out under anesthesia by Indian hemp (laparotomy, thoracotomy and cranial trepanation)." [11]

---

11 Prof. Pierre Huard and Dr. Ming Wong. *Chinese Medicine.* World University Press, London. UK. (p.89).

Jivaka was a great Indian surgeon and famous acupuncturist as described by Dr. Omura:

"In ancient India there was a similar treatment to acupuncture or moxibustion and even treatment by massage as well. In the old texts of Buddhism, the words acupuncture and moxibustion appeared sporadically, and the famous physician of India, Giba [Jivaka] is said in one of the texts such as the Chikitsa Vidya to have been born with an acupuncture needle in the right hand and a drug container in the left hand in about the 5th century B.C." [12]

It was Buddhism that spread the knowledge of Ayurveda and siravedhana acupuncture abroad.

"This highly developed knowledge of medicine [Ayurveda] received patronage of kings. Thereafter, the time came when ambassadors went to East Asian countries, including Ceylon and Indonesia. Amongst them were some Buddhist monks who preached and practiced the Ayurvedic system of medicine. They developed the 'Marma Chikitsa' and it was recognized as Acupuncture." [13]

Tibetan medicine has traditionally also used Ayurvedic medicine according to Tibetan Dr. Yeshi Donden, the chief physician to the Dalai Lama:

"The Tibetan system, mainly derived from ancient Indian Buddhist medicine centers around restoring the three humors Wind[Vata], Bile [Pitta], and Phlegm [Kapha]." [14]

Tibetan medicine has also used Indian acupuncture as mentioned in the Fourth Shastra of the canon and as explained below by Dr. Donden:

"Last, [in the Fourth Shastra] is a section dealing with accessory therapy, these include Moxibustion, Acupuncture, Surgery and so forth." [15]

A needle made of wood could splinter easily when trying to suture a wound, stone obviously provided a stronger alternative. Needles were then fashioned out of stone but this was fine when needles were crude and large, but as ancient technology grew, stone needles became unsuitable as they provided no flexibility to the needle and could only be ground down to a limited extent, before it cracked.

It would not have taken long for humans to figure out that the very animal which they had killed for food, could provide a perfect needle. It was strong

---

12 Dr. Yoshiaki Omura. MD. *Acupuncture Medicine- Its Historical and Clinical Background.* Japan Publications. Japan. (p.15).
13 Dr. D.G.Thatte. *Acupuncture Marma and other Asian Therapeutic Techniques.* Chaukhambha Orientalia, Delhi. 1988. (p.v.)
14 Dr. Yeshi Donden.MD. *Health Through Balance,* Snowlion Publishers. NY. 1986. (p.25).
15 *Ibid.*

and flexible and could be filed or trimmed to a very small diameter and short length indeed. It was the animal bone which remained as a necessary waste by-product which then provided not only a source of needle material but also a source of weapon material, e.g. a knife or axe blade.

Later, needles in India were also fashioned out of bamboo, which were strong, flexible and could be made into thin, sharp instruments for needling. Metal needles soon followed.

> "The science of acupuncture has its roots in the Vedas. The first reference of acupuncture is found in Rig-Veda and at that time separate text was available which was known as 'Suchi Veda'. Bamboo or wooden Suchi- needles were used for acupuncture. During ancient times needles made of wood were used, later on various metal needles were used for this purpose." [16]

According to experts, some of these needles have been found in the ancient site of Takshashila University (Taxilla), India.

> "It is interesting to note that acupuncture was practiced in India in ancient times. Taxilla [acupuncture] needles of different sizes and made up of iron, copper and bronze have been found." [17]

Knowledge Development

Concurrently to all this knowledge, another form of knowledge developed. That was the observation of the Laws of Nature and how they affected living beings. Constant observation of recurrent phenomena led to the realization of existence of factors which could not be seen but nevertheless were real. One of these was the observation that through breathing, 'good' air could be taken in and 'bad' air expelled in order to maintain health.

Although the air could not be seen, it was easy to prove that it was there and necessary, simply by covering the mouth and nose with the hand. Various basic laws were observed, catalogued into the human computer (brain) and then passed down from generation to generation by the spoken word. This was an early form of Science which although limited by a crude technology was not limited in its application and practice. The technology in 50 years time from today will no doubt demonstrate our technology as crude. The word Science itself (scientia) actually means 'to know' and that was exactly what humans were trying to do.

---

16 Drs. Subhash Ranade, Avinash Lele and David Frawley. *Secrets of Marma.* International Academy of Ayurveda Publishing, Pune India. (p.11).
17 Dr. C.L. Nagpal, *Modern Acupuncture.* IATRI, Jaipur, India. (pp.3, 4).

Another discovery was the existence of sensitive or painful spots on the body which appeared to coincide with a dysfunction in the person's health. When the pain spots had disappeared, the dis-ease had similarly banished. Today, Science calls this phenomenon 'referred pain' and nerve 'trigger points' where certain areas of the body reflect pain due to an imbalance or problem in an internal organ. For instance according to current scientific knowledge a liver disorder can refer pain to the area of the right shoulder, although the liver itself is physically nowhere near the pain area. A particular tooth exhibiting pain can indicate a possible problem in the heart.

Eventual cataloguing of these spots led to the realization of internal connections. A painful point in the foot could disappear with the parallel removal of discomfort or pain in the kidneys (urinary system). For instance, painful urination was healed concurrently with the removal of pain in a point on the foot or even a point in the ear.

So, connections between internal organs and external areas of the body were observed and recorded forming a holistic view of the body and providing an understanding of how it could be healed.

Healing could be achieved by various means, perhaps by massaging of the area which was painful, applying certain herbs to the area or else by puncturing the area with a needle. Practical experience over perhaps hundreds or thousands of years led to a strong conviction of the value of using these techniques in certain points and their certain, eventual therapeutic effect.

Exactly which part of the world the above techniques and knowledge first developed is today impossible to say. There is no substantial proof to show this, only hearsay. Each culture and country would attempt to prove that they were the ones who invented or practiced certain things, however as proved by the controversy of martial arts as more and more documentary evidence is gained, less and less certainty develops.

India
The knowledge and practice of the healing descriptions above can nevertheless be shown to have been in existence in India more than 7000 years ago.

According to Ayurvedic expert and author, Dr. C. Thakkur:

> "In the Indian medical classics, known as the Vedas, said to be
> written about 7000 years ago, we find 'Needle Therapy' mentioned there.
> One volume of the Vedas, known as the Suchi Veda, translated as 'the art
> of piercing with a needle' [science of needle therapy] was written about
> 3000 years ago and deals entirely with acupuncture.

Indians have both body acupuncture and ear acupuncture. In the former, they have points (known as Marma: said to heal or kill) which they either burn with a herb, massage or pierce with various types of needles [acupuncture]. The methods are essentially the same [or similar] to those used by the Chinese." [18]

In fact it is in the very ancient Indus Valley Civilization that traces of early medicine, martial arts and yoga can be found. This knowledge led to the development of acupuncture in India where bone or bamboo needles were first used to puncture a pressure point in order to balance energy and cure disease. According to existing evidence, India was probably the most advanced of all the ancient countries in the practice of surgery. It is believed that the practice of acupuncture emerged from the practice of surgical techniques where needles were used by the Indian surgeons. The Vedas are the ancient Indian texts which record this evidence and in which 'needle therapy' (acupuncture) is mentioned.

Later, when metals such as gold, silver and bronze were discovered and freely available, needles were manufactured from these. Their application would depend on the type of metal and nature of the disease, as each metal has distinct features and effects.

Acupuncture was used in India in ancient times and some scholars believe it was due to the unavailability of herbs in Northern India, near the very cold slopes of the Himalayas where no herbs generally grow that the practice of acupuncture began:

"Some scholars believe that acupuncture probably evolved in prehistoric times out of the modifications of the principles of Ayurveda, near the snowy bleaks of the Himalayas [North India], where no herbs were available." [19]

This is an interesting point because the ancient *rishis* or great seers who were meant to have developed Ayurveda were also regarded to have lived in the North of India, at the foot of the Himalayas.

Of course, Ayurvedic acupuncture was later (from about 300 BC) also practiced by the Sri Lankans and later still, by the Tibetans who also received Indian culture via Buddhism. It is believed that the Buddhist concept of non-violence (*ahimsa*) meant that surgery (anatomical dissection) became undesirable but allowed acupuncture to flourish as it does not produce anatomical dissection, unlike surgery.

The great ancient Indian universities of Nalanda and Takshashila are attributed as learning centers not only of Ayurvedic medicine, but also of Ayurvedic acupuncture.

18 Dr. Chandrashekhar Thakkur . *The Ear, Gateway To Balancing The Body.* By Dr. Wexu, M. Aurora Press, Santa Fe, NM (1985). (p.187).
19 Prof. Dr. Sir Anton Jayasuriya. (1994). *Clinical Acupuncture.* B. Jain Publishers. New Delhi, India. (p.369).

Ayurvedic Acupuncture

Indian acupuncture (*Suchi karma*) is termed Ayurvedic acupuncture because the essential knowledge required to use and understand this system has the same basic origins and features as the system used in India, called Ayurveda. It utilizes the same concepts of energies, humors, elements, organs and tissues. They also share the same forms of diagnoses and understand the world and Nature in the same way. So it is therefore acceptable to term this form of acupuncture 'Ayurvedic acupuncture'. Also, Ayurvedic Surgery (*Salya Tantra*) is one of the eight recognized subjects or recorded branches of Ayurveda, acupuncture being a related discipline or sub-branch of this subject.

Suchi Karma

Ayurvedic acupuncture is traditionally also called *Suchi Chikitsa* and also '*BhedanKarma*'.

Suchi Chikitsa literally means 'needle treatment' (whereas karma means 'therapy') and forms part of the broader system called *Marma Chikitsa* (*marma* treatment) of which Indian acupressure-type massage and moxibustion (*agni-karma*) also form part. *Marma Chikitsa* is a generic term for all therapies which treat the *marmas* or Ayurvedic pressure points.

BhedanKarma literally means 'piercing-through therapy' and has a close relative in Ayurvedic surgery (*Salya Tantra*) where it is called *VedhanKarma* (puncturing therapy). *BhedanKarma* (piercing-through therapy) demonstrates the ancient concept that through correct needling (acupuncture), *Prana* or life energy can pierce-through from the macrocosm (universe) to the microcosm (body) via the skin in order to create internal balance or harmony (health).

Ayurvedic acupuncture, being a part of Ayurvedic Science must be enhanced and allowed to grow. The concept of any science is to further research and expand existing knowledge with new knowledge which remains in keeping with the original. Ayurvedic Medicine cannot remain today only as it was once practiced in India. As a living science, it must be adapted to circumstances and locations where it is now practiced and must be enhanced with acceptable knowledge.

Today, Ayurvedic Acupuncturists/ Marmapuncturists (Suchika) and Marma specialists in India are for the most part practitioners of traditional Indian Martial Arts (e.g. Kalari) who generally jealously guard their systems from outsiders.

> *"Though the practical application of the knowledge of body marmas has disappeared from most of India, it persists [mainly] in the southern state of Kerala, among practitioners of the martial art known as Kalari-ppayattu."* [20]

---

20 Svoboda R., *Ayurveda, Life, Health and Vitality*, Arkana Publishers, USA. (p.65).

They are in a minority principally for two reasons:

A) Their traditional upbringing encourages them to keep the system within their own families as a form of trade secret (it is one way of earning a leaving).

B) Past experiences where traditional practitioners had been betrayed by beaurocrats who had promised to give them financial compensation, credit and recognition for their system but once taught, had claimed the system as their own without even a mention of the traditional doctors' contributions.

> *"Today only a few Ayurvedic practitioners have even been*
> *exposed to svarodaya and while many learn the doctrine*
> *of marma while in college, few make use of it in practice."* [19]

Ayurveda in Sri Lanka

Nevertheless, Ayurvedic acupuncture is not only practiced in India today, but is also found in Sri-Lanka (about 50 km from India), where it is well recognized. The Sri-Lankan system of acupuncture is also Ayurvedic acupuncture, since their medical system is also Ayurvedic.

> *"In the Ayurvedic systems of India and Sri Lanka, there are*
> *three pulse positions at each wrist , called vat [Vata],*
> *pith [Pitta] and sem [Kapha]."* [21]

> *" Acupuncture and moxibustion have been used in many*
> *other regions of the world since pre-historic times. It was well*
> *developed in North India and in Sri Lanka before the Christian era."* [22]

> *"From prehistoric times, acupuncture and moxibustion*
> *have been practiced together as complementary forms of therapy,*
> *often on the same patient. In Sri Lanka too, these modalities were closely*
> *related and acupuncture-moxibustion is called vidum- pilissum."* [23]

70% of Sri Lanka's population are Buddhist who originally emigrated from India or were natives converted to Indian Buddhism, while the majority of the remaining people are related to the South Indian Tamils. King Ashoka's son Mahinda is credited with the establishment of Buddhism in Sri Lanka. Especially through Buddhism, Sri Lanka is believed to have inherited Ayurvedic acupuncture (*Vidum*) and Moxibustion (*Pilissum*). *Vidum* means to pierce with a needle or nail etc. In fact, the only specie of Moxa (herb which is burnt to perform moxibustion- heat therapy) found in Sri Lanka is believed to have been imported from India, where today 27 species are found [24].

21 Prof. Dr. Anton Jayasuriya *Clinical Acupuncture*. B.Jain Pub, India. (p.369).
22 Prof. Dr. Anton Jayasuriya *Clinical Acupuncture*. B.Jain Pub, India. (p.17).
23 *Ibid.* (p.707).
24 *Ibid.* (p.709).

Moxa (*artemisia vulgaris*) is called *Nagadamani* in Sanskrit.

According to Prof. Dr. Anton Jayasuriya, instruments used in Sri Lanka for surgery and acupuncture anesthesia about 2400 years ago still exist and in fact surgery with acupuncture anesthesia was carried out at the King Pandukabhaya Hospital in Sri Lanka (500 BC.) [25]. Obviously, the close relationship between India and Sri Lanka for thousands of years, meant that these procedures were likewise carried out in India, as well as in Sri Lanka.

"Be mindful of what the pulse reveals Before thou doest apply The needle science of Iswara ;[God] Revealed in the days gone by.

(From an ancient Sri Lankan ola manuscript, circa 300 BC.)." [26]

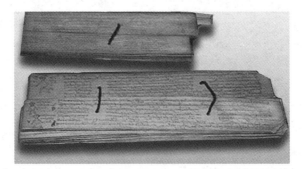

***Fig 3**. Ancient Sri Lankan OLA manuscript depicting Marmapuncture*

It is interesting to note that the above script not only accentuates the use of acupuncture but also Ayurvedic pulse diagnosis in Sri Lanka and India since at least 300 BC.

Ayurvedic Acupuncture in the Sushruta Samhita

Ayurvedic acupuncture is the modern term to denote and differentiate between the Ayurvedic system of acupuncture and other forms such as Chinese, Japanese, and symptomatic treatment (modern medical) acupuncture.

In ancient India, Sushruta, an ancient surgeon and author (about 500 BC) used a form of acupuncture based on Ayurvedic principles, which were also based on the system of Shalya Chikitsa, believed older than Sushruta. He called this system *Siravedhana* (also *siravedhanam*) and described it in his authoritative text, the *Sushruta Samhita*. Sushruta taught *Siravedhana* at the Dhanvantari School of surgery.

---

25 Prof. Dr. Anton Jayasuriya *Clinical Acupuncture*. Medicina Alternativa International, SriLanka. 15th Edition. (p.757).
26 Prof. Dr. Anton Jayasuriya. *Clinical Acupuncture* . B.Jain Pub, India. (p.363).

According to Ayurvedic expert Prof. Dr. H.S. Sharma:

"Siravedhanam and Marma Chikitsa were very prevalent and highly accepted therapies during RgVeda and AtharvaVeda and flourished during Samhita period. Finally, it will be clear to the whole world that Acupuncture [Siravedhana], as we understand today is one of the components of age-old Shalya Chikitsa and is the Indian study of the Dhanvantari School ." [27]

Sushruta's work survived, despite the many invasions of India and the destruction of many places of learning including the former University of Nalanda, considered containing thousands of books on virtually every subject known at that time.

Gradually, as traditional doctors disclose some of their concepts that have been taught by word of mouth for thousands of years after Sushruta, we have begun to understand the wide range of meanings that are traditionally attributed to a particular word or term.

The Sushruta Samhita, written text and attributed to Sushruta is no exception. Scholars have begun to decipher some of the deeper meanings behind many of the terms in this text. What we have recently discovered is a lot of knowledge, specifically on surgery (*Shalya Chikitsa*) and acupuncture.

Sira

The Sanskrit word *sira* has usually been translated as simply 'vein'.

Dr. Joshi explains that:

"Fixed misconceptions reigned and ruined the great science of Ayurveda, and also non- availability of diagrams and illustrations were also responsible for this. This is the reason why even today Dhamani and Sira are interpreted wrongly as blood carrying Artery and Vein." [28]

"Dhamanis (Channels) and Siras (points above dhamanis)." [29]

"Rasa [Prana] is circulated in the dhamanis and there are seven hundred siras embedded in these dhamanis." [30]

Therefore, when someone unfamiliar with the subject translates "puncturing a sira" it can easily be translated as simply "bloodletting", a process by which a vein is punctured to release blood for therapeutic purposes. Actually

---

27 Drs. B.K.Joshi, R.L.Shah, G.Joshi. *Vedic Health Care System.* (Foreword).
28 Joshi et al. (Preface).
29 *Ibid.* (p.42).
30 *Ibid.* (p.1).

'bloodletting' is called *rakta moksha* and not siravedhana but when performing acupuncture, sometimes a few drops of blood are released by the body as a therapeutic reaction- not unlike the healing reaction of raktamoksha. However, the term sira also means a tubular structure allowing flow [sru]. [31]

Joshi explains the word sira as

> *"Sira: Ends, Heads, a Stream."* [32]

Sira can, therefore, be interpreted and translated into a point on the surface of the skin, or acupuncture point.

This *sira* is very much like a fine tube that connects the outer skin with a final destination in a deeper channel (dhamani) and along which the energy known as Prana or Rasa (subtle) flows.

Piercing the entry point on the skin with a needle, we can stimulate this small channel (*sira*) that connects to the deepest channel (*dhamani*) and which eventually stimulates other organic structures (e.g. heart, liver, etc.) through *Prana* or subtle *Rasa*, (*Param Sukshma Rasa*).

Dhamani

The word *dhamani* has usually been translated simply as artery and therefore whose function is to transport blood. *Sushruta* defined *dhamani* (and *sira*) as the channel carrying *Rasa*, the micro nutrient that is currently invisible and is traditionally called *Prana*, Ki or Chi in the East.

In fact, *Sushruta* referred to *Rasa* instead of *Prana* in the context of life energy, so as not to confuse it with the energy moving inward (*prana Vayu*) and mental strength (e.g. *Prana*, *Tejas* and *Ojas*).

The Sanskrit dictionary explains dhamani as

> *"[a]tube (especially) a channel in the human body."* [33]

According to the Sushruta Samhita,

> *"Sutra Sthana 14 and Sharira Sthana 9, it is the Rasa*
> *which flows in the Dhamani and not the blood."* [34]

> *"The finest essence of four types of food we take, flows through*
> *these dhamanis, the Chinese call it as Qi [Prana], and Acharya Sushruta*
> *calls it as Param Sukshma Rasa (ultramicroscopic live force)"* [35]

---

31 Monier - Williams, *English Sanskrit Dictionary*. (p.1217).
32 Joshi *et al.* (p.165).
33 Monier - Williams, *English Sanskrit Dictionary*. (p.510).
34 Joshi *et al.*, (Preface).
35 *Ibid.* (p.4).

The dhamanis are

> "not synonyms of Arteries but Dhamanis are meridians or channels.
> According to Sushruta Sutra sthana 14/3." [36]

Therefore, the channels or meridians are invisible dhamanis connecting with key structures such as the liver or the kidneys and by which therapeutically one can influence the functioning of these organs.

Sushruta explains that there are 24 dhamanis in the human body which are associated with various organs, although there are only 12 recognized organs (liver, kidney, heart, etc.). This is because each organ has two associated channels, one that flows through the left side and one that flows through the right side of the body, such that each organ influences both sides of the human body and there are therefore 24 dhamanis, two for each organ.

> "According to Sushruta there are twenty-four Dhamanis." [37]

Nadis

The word *Nadi* meaning a hollow tube or pipe has always been thought to describe the channels that carry prana or life force to various structures such as the *marmas*. Currently, we can understand that the *dhamanis* are forms of *nadis* and these are referred to as *dhamanis* by *Sushruta*. The *dhamanis* normally connect and interact with the 12 organs of the body. Each organ has a *dhamani* on each side of the body. For example, the heart has a channel in the left arm and a channel in the right arm, both of which are connected together in the Heart.

In this book, the two terms, *nadis* and *dhamanis* are generally interchangeable. All are forms of *nadis* but not all *dhamanis* are called *nadis*. However, to be technically accurate, the *nadis* often refer to the meridians that carry prana to the 107 *marmas* and the chakras *as well* as the sense organs (e.g. organ of sight), while *dhamanis* refer to the meridians that carry prana to approximately 700 *siras* or acupuncture points (some of which are in areas of *marma*) inserted in its corresponding *dhamani* or meridian, and which eventually allows prana to flow into or out of their corresponding organ (e.g. liver).

The two additional channels or meridians are known as the Conception Vessel (C) [*Artava Nadi*] or Conception channel and the Governing Channel (G) [*Shukra Nadi*] or Minister channel. These vessels are not directly related to any of the twelve organs and are called *nadis* instead of *dhamanis*. This is probably

---

36 *Ibid.* (p.3).
37 Joshi et al. (p.4).

due to the delegation of importance, namely, that the interactions of the *nadis* are seen as more complex than the *dhamanis*, perhaps more important as they directly relate to the chakras or energy vortices. Furthermore, the flow through the organ channels is circular and of a closed loop, while the flow through the Conception and Governing nadis are separate and also of a closed circuit of their own.

Marmas

The *marmas* are large accumulation centers of *prana*, besides being much more susceptible areas to trauma and injury. The marmas always contain one or more *siras*, while the *siras* do not always relate to one of the 107 *marmas*. Some marmas have the same sira in common. It can be perhaps argued that all siras are in fact marmas, perhaps micro marmas unless they are in the direct location of one of the 107 marmas or zones.

Sushruta treated many wounded warriors with lethal injuries to the *marmas*, hence their willingness to ensure that marmas were not injured not only in battle but also during surgery or other invasive therapies.

Therefore, the *marmas* are specific body areas or zones and are more susceptible to injury, while the siras are tube-shaped structures that carry Prana from the *dhamanis* or internal network of meridians to the skin on the outer surface of the body, where they terminate in a small specific area, a head or point. It is this point that is punctured in Ayurvedic acupuncture.

Dr. Frawley explains:

> *"While the smaller marmas can be called 'points' the larger marmas are more accurately described as 'regions' or 'zones'."* [38]

These points are called 'siras', and the regions or vital zones are called '*marmas*' (containing one or more *siras*).

It is interesting to note that in south of India, in the ancient textbooks known as Tamil Marma Shastras, the term sira is often considered as a synonym of marma, according to expert Dr. Thatte. [39]

Conclusion

Bri. Maya Tiwari describes the role of acupuncture in Ayurvedic marma therapy as:

> *"to stimulate, repair and heal these vital points by Ayurvedic acupuncture."* [40]

---

38 Drs. Ranade, Lele and Frawley. *Ayurveda and Marmatherapy.* (pp.30-31).
39 Dr.D.G.Thatte. *Acupuncture Marma and other Asian Therapeutic Techniques.* Chaukhambha Orientalia, Delhi. 1988. (p.23)
40 Tiwari, M., *Ayurveda Secrets of Healing.* Lotus Press, USA. 1997.

As our world moves toward a global system of international medicine instead of folk medicine system, adaptation of Ayurveda and Ayurvedic acupuncture will become important pillars for its essential development. As an important part of this system Ayurvedic practitioners can improve the overall health using this ancient but modern science of natural health.

The purpose of any science is to investigate and expand original existing knowledge by adding new ones. Ayurvedic medicine today cannot remain as it was practiced in ancient India. As a living science, it must be adapted to the circumstances and the places where its practice is needed, enhancing it with acceptable knowledge.

'We must improve and facilitate the growth of Ayurvedic acupuncture as it is a valuable part of Ayurvedic Science'.

Philosophy of ayurvedic acupuncture

Traditional Philosophy

Ayurvedic acupuncture inherits its philosophy from the Ayurvedic system of medicine and surgery. Acupuncture is therefore related to these other methods of healing and depends on the same core of knowledge as these others. As needle therapy (which is what acupuncture is traditionally called) is an adjunct or co-therapy to Ayurvedic treatment, so it is viewed in the same light.

It utilizes the same view of the cosmos and the human body and diagnoses and treats in much the same manner as other Ayurvedic treatments. Whether a practitioner prescribes an herb or indeed provides needle therapy for the patient, the methodology is identical although the materials or vehicles are different.

Herbs attempt to balance the humoral energies (Tridoshas) via ingestion or application on the skin. Acupuncture attempts this same balancing act via needling various body points (*marmas*) which stimulate the healing mechanisms and balance the humoral energies. Where acupuncture differs from the former therapy is in that the direct effect on the body which later affects the humors, is provided by manipulation of the Pranic energy or life force, via the needle. Dried herbs have lost this life force energy (*Prana*) and thus they mainly function via direct effects on the humors, through their heating (e.g. chillies), cooling (e.g. slippery elm), drying (e.g. rhubarb) or moistening (e.g. watermelon) actions on the body. Obviously, if the herbs are taken fresh, that is still containing much of the energy (*Prana*), then this effect would be somewhat akin to acupuncture. This is why Ayurveda recommends the ingestion of fresh food (which is also a medicine) which should contain *Prana*.

The philosophy of Ayurvedic acupuncture relates that through needling various locations on the body, a therapeutic reaction occurs either locally or remote to the location where the needle is inserted. These sensitive points which are found to have very low galvanic skin resistance are called *marmas* and siras and are located all over the human body. Modern research has discovered many more *marmas/siras* than were previously used or known. An electronic device called an acupuncturescope (acuscope), can detect and locate these *marmas/siras*.

The sensitive points themselves are linked by a yet unseen system of invisible channels (nadis) which themselves carry *Prana*, the life energy. These channels deliver energy to the *marmas* or points with which they relate. These points are generally high energy concentrations of *Prana*. As will be seen later in this book, the sensitive points which traditionally are called marmas also include other points called *siras* and the nadis are also classified into two, *nadis* and *dhamanis*.

Each major organ in the body (as classified in Ayurveda) has one of these channels or Pranic artery which provide connections between the relevant *marmas* (and siras) and the appropriate organ located in the torso (e.g. the heart). By needling points along the related channel, the organ can be made to improve in function, in itself a therapeutic or homoeostatic action.

Ayurveda diagnoses a patient according to well established guidelines. These forms of guidelines allow the acupuncturist to ascertain the correct organ which is unbalanced and thereby treat the needling points in the corresponding channel.

One of the major philosophical principles is the knowledge of the Five Elements (ether, wind, fire, water, earth) which assist the proper application of therapy by aligning the correct diagnosis with the correct organ or channel treatment. For instance an excess in Fire may result in excitability (fire in excess), its needling treatment may be in a point on the heart channel (H7) since the heart is generally aligned with Fire.

The uniqueness of Ayurveda is also the development of three humoral energies (themselves generated from the Five Elements) which likewise furthers the potential of the diagnoses and treatments by recognizing each person as an individual, aligned to one of these three energies.

It is the person's connection with one of these three energies which dictates the way the person, acts, feels, looks and reacts to medication. These energies when aggravated cause imbalances, directly recognizable and aligned with the three humors.

Needle therapy (Suchi karma) (or BhedanKarma) is an effective and ancient form of prevention as well as therapy. It requires simple apparatus and its effectiveness is well documented by modern Science.

Scientific Explanations for Acupuncture

Currently, there are many scientific theories on why and how acupuncture works, the major ones are described below.

Acupuncture's Major Effects:

(a) Analgesia

(b) Sedation

(c) Homoeostasis

(d) Immune system enhancement

(e) Anti-inflammatory

(f) Anti-allergic

(g) Psychological tranquillizing action

(h) Recovery of motor system disorders.

Gate Control Theory of Pain
(Melzack & Wall 1965)

Large diameter nerve fibers conduct nerve impulses excluding pain and are myelinated.

Small diameter nerve fibers conduct pain impulses in the nervous system and are unmyelinated.

Large Diameter fibers are divided into A and B type fibers.

A Fibers have fast conduction (130 m/sec) and are generally involved in life-threatening nerve impulses.

B Fibers have medium speed conduction (10 m/sec) and are generally involved in conduction of non life-threatening impulses.

Both A and B type fibers conduct touch, pressure, heat and cold as well as position of joints impulses through the nervous system.

Small diameter fibers or C Fibers have slow conduction (0.5 m/sec) and usually conduct pain impulses from the skin and visceral nerves.

In the Gate Control theory, the small diameter fibers open the gate for pain transmission (allow painful impulses through) while the large diameter fibers under acupuncture action, send a major stream of non-painful nerve impulses to the gate, jamming it shut and preventing the small diameter fibers from connecting and thereby preventing the pain impulses from getting through.

Chemical/ Humoral Mechanisms

Acupuncture releases various chemical transmitters in order to bind with the opiate receptors found in the neurons (nerve cells) of the nervous system. These opiate receptors cause analgesic effects on the body when a chemical (natural or otherwise) joins the receptor. In the case of Enkephalins released by the midbrain, this chemical binds with the receptor, causing analgesia. In the case of morphine or one of the artificial derivatives (*valium*) these chemicals cause similar analgesic reactions by binding to the receptors. Endorphins are natural chemical transmitters produced in the pituitary gland which are also released under acupuncture treatment. Endorphins are nevertheless at least twenty times more powerful in analgesic effect than morphine and thus the success rate of acupuncture in the treatment of pain.

Thalamic Neuron Theory

The Thalamic Neuron theory states that acupuncture points are effective because the same locations of points in the body are found in the thalamus, as if in a fetal position. Consequently, needling of an acupuncture point causes an appropriate reaction in the related part of the thalamus which is then transmitted elsewhere for action (therapeutic effect).

None of these theories, separately or combined totally explain the concept of acupuncture and why it works. There are obviously many more sophisticated mechanisms as yet unknown to Science, which allow acupuncture's success in the treatment of many diseases as well as management of pain and other debilitating effects. In order to ascertain how acupuncture can be totally explained scientifically, Science itself is being modified from within, into a more holistic and humanistic system (e.g. quantum physics etc.)

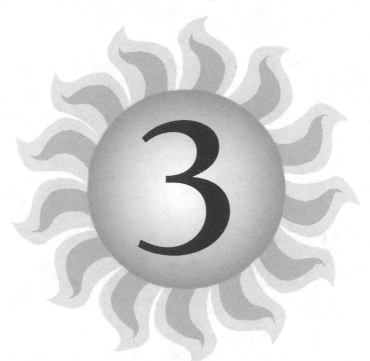

3 Energetics of ayurveda

Prana- the subtle energy

The system of Ayurvedic acupuncture, like Ayurveda itself is totally reliant on *Prana*, the subtle form of energy that keeps all living things healthy and alive.

Prana is a subtle type of bio-energy that Dash explains is the "life-force or *elan vital*." [41] This life-force keeps the person or living being alive and is similarly found in plants. In fact, by ingesting fresh plants (vegetables, fruit etc.) the person is also ingesting *Prana* which is then absorbed in the body to perform its life-keeping function. *Prana* also enters the body via the breath, since its Sanskrit root is *an-* to breathe.

Dr. Lad explains that:

"Prana or life energy enters the body through breath taken in through the nose." [42]

Svoboda explains that:

"You receive Prana, the life-force from both air and food. Your system will feel less hunger if your breathing is good because it can rely less on food for its Prana." [43]

41 Dash, B. (p.156).
42 Lad, V. (p.75).
43 Svoboda, R. *Prakruti, Your Ayurvedic Constitution.* (p.94).

Consequently, food that has been irradiated or microwaved tends to have a deficiency of *Prana* since it has been dissipated by the process of these types of cooking. Obesity can therefore be caused by an insufficiency of *Prana* in foods (e.g. processed foods) since the person needs to eat more for compensation.

After it enters the body, *Prana* circulates through various subtle channels called *nadis*, later entering the *dhamanis* or organ meridians and *siras* or points/miniature channels (not unlike arterioles or capillaries extending from the arteries until they reach the skin surface) and is then able to control, stimulate and keep alive the living organism.

Iyengar explains:

"The Nadis [bio-energy channels] penetrate the body from the soles of the feet to the crown of the head... in them is Prana, the breath of life." [44]

Iyengar then further explains:

"Prana is the energy permeating the universe at all levels.
It is physical, mental, intellectual, sexual, spiritual and cosmic energy.
All vibrating energies are Prana. The prime mover of all activity.
It is energy which creates, protects and destroys." [45]

Consequently, *Prana* is the underlying force or impetus of all living beings and is required for life to be sustained.

According to Feuerstein, *Prana* assumes five distinct functions after it enters the body:

"(1) Prana - draws life-force into the body;
(2) Apana - expels life-force;
(3) Vyana - distributes and circulates the life-force;
(4) Samana - takes care of the assimilation of food;
(5) Udana- responsible for the production of speech." [46]

Dr. Frawley explains that:

"all material energy is a development of pure energy,
which is the power of life itself." [47]

So Prana is involved in every human function or mechanism. In fact, it is the matrix on which the other Ayurvedic energies of Tridoshas (three humors) and the Five Elements (*Pancha Mahabhutas*) are built.

---

44 Iyengar, B.K.S. (p.32).
45 *Ibid.*(p.12).
46 Feuerstein, G. (p.162).
47 Frawley, D. (p.3).

In ancient Ayurveda, the pure energy (*Prana*) and pure consciousness (Purusha) were regarded as inter-twined and interrelated, and both contained within the same vehicle into the body.

As Frawley also states:

"Hidden in all energy is the working of a conscious will. Hence this Prana was also called Purusha, the Primal Spirit." [48]

Purusha can be affected by the wrong or right ideas and psychological or spiritual actions, which can nevertheless direct the body either into disease or health.

Charaka testifies to this fact when he distinctly discerns between Purusha and *Prana* as he considers Purusha different from the "six elements" (Five Elements + *Prana*) which nevertheless evolve from Purusha:

"Purusha comprises six dhatus (elements) viz. five Mahabhutas (in their subtle form) and consciousness." [49]

Charaka, being influenced by Samkhya philosophy considered consciousness as part of *Prana* and *Prana* as part of consciousness (soul?) in keeping with the religious connotations upheld at the time.

Such is the importance of *Prana* according to Lad:

"[that it]…governs all higher cerebral activities. The function of mind, memory, thought and emotions are all under the control of Prana." [50]

Consequently, *Prana* is involved in psychosomatic diseases as well as in normal physical maladies. Treatment of *Prana* can therefore treat psychological diseases as well.

Prana has its equivalent in the Chinese and oriental concepts of Chi, and as Dr. Svoboda explains:

"Prana is the life force, equivalent to the chi or ki in Oriental medicine." [51]

Since *Prana* is essentially obtained from breathing and carried by oxygen molecules, then it is logical to use breathing exercises to correctly control *Prana*. But this is only one way of doing so, since *Prana* can also be controlled in the body via acupuncture or indeed any therapeutic / prophylactic system that controls and affects Pranic energy flow. In consequence, Marma Chikitsa (also *chikilsa*) of which acupuncture and *marma* massage form part can also be considered as a form of subtle *Pranayama*.

48 *Ibid.*
49 Sharma R. and Dash, B. *Charaka Samhita.*Vol.2 (p.314).
50 Lad, V. (p.109).
51 Svoboda, R. Prakruti, *Your Ayurvedic Constitution.* (p.123).

Prana

Ayurvedic acupuncture is basically an energy-based system, which views all things as a true manifestation of energy (*Prana*), which itself may be derived from pure consciousness (*Avyakta*) (from the joining of *Purusha*-universal conscious element and *Prakruti*- primordial matter).

The human body is in fact reflections of the Universe and via the energy, all living things develop.

Ayurvedic acupuncture's aim is to bring into balance the disharmony of the body (microcosm) and into line with the harmony of the Universe (macrocosm). This is achieved by manipulation of the energy via the acupuncture needle (*suchi*) inserted at strategic points called siras which are embedded into meridians referred to as dhamanis. The resultant internal reaction in the body results in health or balance (homoeostasis).

Life Energy

Prana is the bio-energy that keeps everything alive and yet its loss will result in death of the living organism. Prana derives from the Sanskrit–*an*, which means 'breath' and so it demonstrates the fact that the bio-energy is carried into the body, principally by the breath or air. Likewise, plants receive this energy via their own breath or air (oxygen is a carrier substance). Later, humans attain *Prana* from these plants which have previously attained it from the air itself.

Prana is the driving force behind every action in the living organism and is the substructure behind all actions in the universe. Through our atmosphere, it is the driving force of Wind (*Vayu*) and the wind energy termed *Vata* in the body.

It appears at the atomic level as well as at the molecular and sub-atomic levels. The movement within the atom (e.g. by the electrons) is related to *Prana* and *Vayu* (wind).

"The Chinese call it Qi (Chi) and Acharya
Sushruta calls it Param Sukshma Rasa." [52]

"The function of Param Suskshma Rasa [prana] is to nourish the body
continuously all the 24 hours [of the day], as kidney meridian nourishes ears while
gall bladder meridian nourishes eyes (see Shringataka Marma, Su.Sharir, 6/27).
This Rasa is responsible for growth, supports the live forces of the body and cures
the diseases. This is essential for treatment. This function is under the subconscious
level and cannot be measured objectively. According to Sushruta, its mechanism of
action cannot be consciously defined." [53]

---

52 Joshi, *et al.* (p.4).
53 Joshi, *et al.* (p.5).

The Five Elements

The Five Physical Energies (*Pancha Mahabhutas*)

Besides *Prana* (energy) there are another five primordial elements which also form part of the underlying cosmic stratum. These five are part of matter (the more physical side of the cosmic equation) and their attributes are progressively physical as considered by Charaka. They are the gaseous, radiant, liquid and solid states of matter, and are represented by Wind (or Air), Fire, Water and Earth respectively. Ether represents the ethereal aspect of matter.

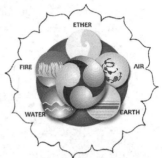

Fig.4. *The Five Elements*

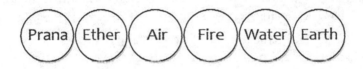

Prana Ether Air Fire Water Earth

All forms of matter contain these additional four elements but in differing ratios so as to give the substance its own particular, recognizable qualities or structure. For instance, a rock logically has a majority of earth but also must have some water in order to provide cohesion between the earth particles. It must also have some fire (perhaps regularly obtained from the Sun) as otherwise the rock would be totally freezing in temperature. But nothing in life is in fact totally solid as outlined by Science, so there are gaps between the various atomic particles, even though generally seen as solid.

The Five Elements

The *Pranic* flow from the subtle realm into our physical sphere, allows a number of elements to develop from the life force, in order to form life. These five elements appear in order of subtleness: Ether, Wind, Fire, Water and Earth. These are called in Ayurveda **The Five Great Elements** (*Pancha Mahabhutas*).

These five elements are initially of a very subtle nature (not able to be seen) and are termed *Tanmatras* (energy quanta), yet with development within Nature, they become more and more physical until we can actually observe them with the human eye. Then, they are termed *Mahabhutas*. These form the material world, but it requires *Prana* also for movement and specifically, life, to be maintained. As an example, there is no doubt that moisture in the air can not be seen, this forms a very subtle form of water. Later, this condenses to form rain or water droplets, which can then be seen.

Each element relates to one or more organs and tissues, but also each element or energy leads to the formation and regulation of additional energies or forces within the body. These include the Three Humoral Energies (*Tridoshas*), Immunity (*Ojas*), Metabolism (*Agni*) and a myriad of other known Ayurvedic factors. *Agni*, for example is *Prana* +Fire.

Ether. *Akasha*: 'Kash', to radiate. That which does not provide resistance.

Ether is the most subtle element and is the primary one. It is the first that interfaces with Prana in the development of the body. It is the space or area (matrix) in which electrons circulate within the atom. Ether also means 'space' and it forms the grid, which allows further building of the body.

The word 'quintessential' has come to mean the ultimate but in reality it means the fifth element or Ether. In marmapunture the ultimate energy is Prana, but it demonstrates how important the ancients considered Ether, as the ultimate element, the basis for matter.

Ether was considered by the ancients as essentially of a gaseous, radiant nature and is not unlike the more physical ether, which is a form of alcohol and anesthetic gas. The alcohol's qualities are:

 (a) cold and drying- Primary qualities
 (b) hot and drying when ignited. Secondary qualities.

So too, the element of Ether (*Akasha*) has these qualities (a) outside the body and (b) inside the body.

As will be noticed later, these qualities greatly direct the body into dis-harmony and also back into harmony, depending on what action has been taken.

Wind. *Vayu*: 'va', movement, oscillation, vibration.

Wind (Air) is the motivator of action or movement, not only of the physical aspects but also of the subtle aspects (e.g. movement of thoughts). Often, a derangement of wind causes either a lack of movement or perhaps exaggerated movement (e.g. tornado). In the body too, this is translated as a lack or excess of movement or action.

Wind (containing *Prana*) is represented by the movement in the atom, especially the electrons. It is the electron(s) that circulates in an orbit-form around the nucleus of the atom.

In the body, Wind has the general qualities of cooling and drying (similar to the primary qualities of Ether). It is involved in the transmission of nerve impulses, in the movement of the joints and muscles, in the circulation of ideas within the brain. It is necessary for any action to take place. The terms Wind and Air are often interchangeable.

Fire. *Tejas*: 'heat', fire or radiation.

Fire is the third most subtle element and is caused by the movement of the primordial particles, resulting in friction or heat. The quality of fire is obviously hot, but is also drying (e.g. Sahara desert) and similar to the Secondary qualities of Ether.

Fire is involved in the 'cooking process' of the cosmos and the microcosm (body). It assists in the shaping of matter into the correct formation. Consider that without the fire/heat, a cake mixture will never develop into a suitable cake.

Fire is also involved in metabolism of the body and in the hormonal system (which requires fire to a great extent). For instance, excess thyroid hormone in the body causes excess metabolism, resulting in weight loss and feeling hotter.

Fire is the potential (or latent) energy that is housed in the atom and if released suddenly it would result in extreme heat (e.g. nuclear explosion).

Water. *Jala*: water, fluid, cohesion, force.

Water (also called *Ap*) is the element that provides the cohesion for the other elements and also allows flow through the body. It assists in transporting nutrients (e.g. blood, plasma) and prevents excessive solidification of the other elements. This would otherwise result in rigidity and lack of movement (a rock).

Water helps to keep the body temperature at the appropriate level and has a major controlling action on Fire. When Water is deficient in the body, this allows dryness and possible rigidity/congestion (blood thickens when water is removed) (similar to the qualities of Wind). Water also helps in flushing out the impurities of the body (toxins) which are produced either as a by-product of cell digestion (endotoxins) or else via absorption of unsuitable material into the body (exotoxins). This is the process of elimination (via the kidneys).

Water is involved in keeping related ideas together in the mind and allows proper flow of thoughts, which may finally develop into an innovation, or invention.

Water is the force or energy of cohesion between the various atomic particles (proton, neutron, and electron) as well as between the individual atoms.

Water is the most common element in the human body and therefore is involved in most activities.

Water is a principal element of the Kapha Dosha (Earth+Water), it is also an important element of the Pitta Dosha (Fire+Water) and is an essential element of the Vata dosha because a lack of Water equates with Vata and elimination (via Water) is a Vata function, especially through the Vata area of the body (below the navel).

Earth. *Prithvi*: offering resistance, solidification, causing congestion.

Earth is the last element of the Five. It is the solid aspect of Nature or solid state of matter. It allows growth and solidity and is necessary for future genesis of living beings. It prevents the body from collapsing as a jelly, as it provides stability. It is involved in the muscular/skeletal system (calcium is an Earth element) which provides a frame for the body.

Earth in excess would provide rigidity to the joints of the body and prevent movement in these. It would allow further weight gain, either muscle or fat or both. It may lead to excess body hair.

Each of the elements, develop from most subtle to most physical in the order described above. Prana winds its way through each one of them and is involved in the whole process.

"Ayurveda regards the human body and its sensory experiences as manifestations of cosmic energy [Prana] expressed in the five elements… these elements sprang from pure Cosmic Consciousness." [54]

The Cycles Of Prana And The Five Elements

Creation/Destruction of Life

Having realized the first stage of creation of the cosmos (according to Charaka and other writers) between *Prana* (energy) and *Akasha* (matter), pure consciousness (Purusha/Chetana) continued its journey towards creating life. This was achieved by creating movement between the energy (*Prana*) and the matter (*Akasha*) particles. This movement was a form of subtle wind (since wind's main characteristic is movement), so it was via motion that the second "physical" element (Wind) evolved. This element is named *Vayu*, which literally means wind. It is also the vehicle via which *Prana* descended all the way from the subtle realm to the physical living universe and into the body. Svoboda mentions that Prana is contained in oxygen molecules and consequently taken into the body via air (wind). [55]

Wind (*Vayu*) via its movement, also caused friction amongst the particles of matter. This friction in turn resulted in heat, Ayurveda calls this heat - Fire (*Tejas* or *Agni*). Fire then melted some of the existing particles that formed a sort of special liquid. This special liquid, considered and forming Water (*Ap*) in Ayurveda, then eventually mixed with the existing matter particles to form a type of mud which eventually solidified or hardened thus forming Earth (*prithvi*).

---

54 Lad, V. 1984. (p.25).
55 Svoboda, R. *Prakruti, Your Ayurvedic Constitution.* (p.124).

The final stage was achieved when earth was formed and life began.

Althroughout, *Prana* was involved and was the mover being the whole process.

Charaka explains:

*"The Soul [that is Prana] unites with the Akasha [ether]
and then with the other four bhutas [elements]
whose attributes are more and more manifested successively."* [56]

The above quote from Charaka essentially means that *Prana* was first, which then joined with *Akasha* (ether) which then joined with the other four elements. These four elements appeared according to how physical they were (manifested). The most physical, (Earth) manifested or came last according to its attributes. It is logical to assume that Earth is much more physical than Water or Fire or Wind or even Ether. In this case, each one in line is more physical (less subtle) than the previous.

Wheel of Creation (Nirmana Chakra)

In Ayurvedic acupuncture this process of creation (via *Prana* and the Five Elements) which has been clearly outlined by Charaka, is traditionally called the Wheel of Creation. This is in accordance with the concept of the Buddhist 'Wheel of Life' (Pali: *bhava chakra*) represented by a cart wheel which Feuerstein explains has *"twelve links."*[57]

The Wheel of Creation is termed *Nirmana chakra* (lit. 'creation wheel') and is represented by a wheel of five links, one for each of the Five Elements. It forms part of a whole therapeutic/diagnostic concept, which is essential for understanding acupuncture, especially from the Ayurvedic perspective.

The Wheel of Creation virtually explains that each element was created out of the previous more subtle element and is found according to the following chart:

ELEMENT		Effect
Prana	Bio-energy	Most subtle
Akasha	Ether	
Vayu	Wind	
Tejas	Fire	
Ap	Water	
Prthvi	Earth	Most physical

56 Sharma R. and Dash B. (p.390).
57 Feuerstein, G. (p.56).

Human Reproduction

The Wheel of Creation is also continuously emulated by human sexual reproduction whereby the process of sex and conception that is human 'creation' is
represented by this wheel.

(1) Firstly, the human male considered to have positive energy is the *Prana*
energy of the Wheel of Creation.

(2) The human female, representing the negative polarity is Ether or matter, the second subtle element in line.

(3) By male and female coition (*Prana* joining with *Akasha*) via a process of
movement- intercourse (Wind)

(4) friction is created (Fire) finally resulting in orgasm

(5) where a reproductive fluid is released- ejaculation (Water) which then
joins the released female reproductive product (ovum)

(6) to form a foetus (Earth). Once the fetus or child matures to an adult,
the whole process re-occurs by the male (*Prana*) joining the female
(*Akasha*) etc in sexual intercourse.

Cycle of Human Creation		
(1) **PRANA**	Male	(+ve)
(2) *Ether*	Female	(-ve)
(3) *Wind*	Coition	(movement)
(4) *Fire*	Orgasm	(friction)
(5) *Water*	Ejaculation	(liquefaction)
(6) *Earth*	Conception	(solidification)

Charaka taught the above cycle of (human) creation, as illustrated in the following quote from his *Samhita* (textbook):

> "*The embryo is formed by the five Mahabhutas (elements) viz. Ether, Wind, Fire,
> Water and Earth and it serves as a receptacle for consciousness. The Soul (i.e.
> conscious element [= Prana]) constitutes the sixth element responsible for the
> formation of the embryo.*" [58]

As Charaka mentioned, the cosmos were created with the soul (*Prana*) first
and each element according to their descending order of subtleness (as quot-
ed above), then *Prana* is obviously regarded first with Ether and the other
elements appearing in the abovementioned order. The sequence of human

---

58 Sharma R. and Dash, B., Vol. 2. (p.388).

sexual reproduction therefore mirrors the Wheel of Creation, since birth after all represents creation.

Wheel of Dissolution

Once the living being which is deteriorating in health finally dies, the process of dissolution commences. Dissolution is translated as meaning death, termination or breaking up into parts (Collins Dictionary). Dissolution then involves the Five Elements breaking up into parts after bodily *Prana* has returned back to the source of energy from where it originated, this is the very most final stage of life.

Feuerstein explains that the process of dissolution of life, according to the Mahanirvana- Tantra (V.93ff) is as follows:

> *"The element earth is dissolved into that of water, water into fire, fire into air [wind] , air into ether, ether into the sense of egoity [= Prana] (ahamkara), that into the 'great' principle (mahat), that into the world-ground (prakruti) and the world-ground into the transcendent Being or Brahman ."* [59]

In effect, the cyclic return of the Five Elements (*Pancha Mahabhutas*) to the Pranic source (via dissolution) is opposite in direction to their cyclic creation. This has the effect of creating a reaction from very physical (Earth) to most subtle (Ether) to then reach the Pranic source. Indian religious philosophy of course, follows *Prana* back to its source, to the Originator (Brahman).

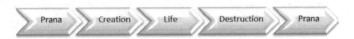

Wheel Of Destruction (Vinasha Chakra)

The Wheel of Dissolution examined above is the physical, structural process by which all forms of matter and energies break up and return to the pure form of energy (also considered as consciousness). There is also another type of wheel which deals with dissolution but in this case is the functional process (disease process) by which the energy returns to its most pure form. This is the Wheel of Destruction (Vinasha Chakra) which outlines the method by which the body progressively destroys itself due to illness or disease, prior to Prana's departure from the body. Although both wheels deal with the elements in the same inter-relationship, the direction of Destruction (disease) however resembles the Wheel of Creation, as the functional process is opposite to the structural process.

---

59 Feuerstein, G. (p.155).

Disease normally starts in an imbalance of *Prana* (subtle) and progressively becomes more and more physical. This essentially means that perhaps a problem started by anxiety (subtle) affecting *Prana* and resulted in a chronic, physical malady such as cancer, over a length of time.

Dr. Kulkarni explains that:

> *"abnormal Vata [=Prana] has been described*
> *a main cause for all diseases in the body."* [60]

Dr. Frawley equates Vata with Prana when he states that:

> *"The term 'Prana' is also used in a broader sense to*
> *indicate Vata in general, as all Vatas derive from it."* [61]

As the disease progresses in seriousness, so it becomes more and more physical. It starts with *Prana* (*Vata*) and ends in Earth, which is the most physical element. The sequence of disease (Wheel of Destruction) when examined then demonstrates the same elements in the same format as the Wheel of Creation.

Both of these wheels are therefore identical since one is the commencement and the other the end of the physical representation of Prana in the cosmos (life). They are both the opposite but normal aspects of life (creation-destruction). Charaka explains this when he states:

> *"The Universe moves around from the unmanifested*
> *stage to the manifested one [creation] and then again*
> *from the manifested stage to the unmanifested one [destruction]."* [62]

PURIFICATION

Elements tend to purify each other. In Ayurvedic acupuncture this purification is also called the Destruction Cycle or wheel. By one element generally destroying (just slightly) the quality of another, it tends to purify it. For instance Water destroys/purifies Earth so that water (flow) checks the function of earth (rigidity) because otherwise the person would not be able to move because of too much earth.

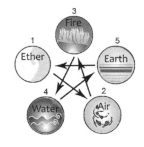

Fig.5. Cycle of Destruction

60 Kulkarni, P.H. (p.9).
61 Frawley, D. (p.7).
62 Sharma, R. and Dash, B. (p.328).

The Cycle of the Elements purifying (destroying) each other are:

1. Ether purifies Wind
2. Wind purifies Fire
3. Fire purifies Water
4. Water purifies Earth
5. Earth purifies Ether

Ether Purifies Wind

Wind (air) when enclosed in a confined space tends to become stale. Ether or space allows air the opportunity to move as the quality of wind is movement. Congestion in the body perhaps caused by blockages in the body channels (srotas, dhamanis and nadis) by excess earth can reduce the space for wind. Increasing space (ether) by unblocking the channels or consuming high ether containing foods (Vata +) can allow air its movement and normal expression.

Wind Purifies Fire

Fire can be destroyed/purified by Wind as in the case of a bushfire and change of direction of the wind which will then snuff it out. Air can also assist in cleaning/ purifying dirty fire (smoke). This is important in the body especially with Agni, in the digestive system (*jatharagni*), liver (*bhuta-agni*) and mental fire (*Tejas*).

Fire Purifies Water

Water can be destroyed/purified by Fire. Sterility (purification) of the water can occur by boiling it (with fire). Excess water can be reduced by boiling also so that Fire destroys the water (but only to a balanced level). When this mechanism works perfectly, there is the right amount of water (or fluid) in the body.

Water Purifies Earth

Earth can be destroyed/purified by Water. If there is excess earth (including Ama) in the body, this tends to dirty it so water can clean or purify it. Imagine a bucket of dirt and then add water. If enough water is added as compensation, the water will go from muddy to murky to clear until all earth seems to have disappeared. Water purifies the channels that have become congested by earth (ama) by applying flow and cleansing the channels.

Earth Purifies Ether

Excess ether can cause expansion in the body by producing too much space. This may be in the form of cysts which are forms of "hollow organs" which then trap fluids. It's interesting that the throat is under the auspices of the Throat

Chakra which is the ether chakra. Often, cysts or abscesses (hollow spaces) can develop in the throat, next to or on the thyroid gland which relates to Ether.

Earth can solidify these hollow spaces. Earth can bring together ether, in the body by constriction.

Elements need to be "destroyed" appropriately so that they do not grow beyond their required levels. For instance, if Earth kept increasing without any form of purification or destruction, then the person would continue to grow in size, muscles would keep growing and fat would keep increasing. Cells are constantly destroyed in the body and new ones take their place as a normal process. This is a form of purification and destruction for positive reasons.

Any of the above elements can also over-purify any other related element which can then cause an imbalance and lead to disease. This becomes real destruction above an acceptable level.

The Other Two Wheels

The process of creation and destruction although very important for life (and eventual death), are obviously not all the processes which exist. Life must continue by processes besides being born or dying, other sequences must also occur. An analogy can be drawn with an automobile. The intention of a manufacturer (or a buyer) of a car is not simply to produce a car and then as soon as it has been "created" then to wreck it (destroy it). Usually, the purpose for the car is to supply transportation to its owner for a certain length of time. In so doing, it provides a sense of satisfaction and also for transportation. But in order to do so, the car must have a brake which slows it down when gaining unwanted speed, this provides a source of control as otherwise the occupant may be involved in an accident. Also, the car must have an accelerator pedal and a fuel tank by which the car can travel forward or backward, by providing fuel to the engine. This provides a source of continuity or support. Water and oil are also required for support. Without these important features in the car, it would not travel.

Likewise, the human body must firstly be created (like the manufacturing of the car), then fuel (food, water) and the correct support must be given to it. But also, there must be a mechanism by which the body can slow itself down or allow itself to speed up as required (brake). This is the process of control and is medically termed 'Homoeostasis' which means to be balanced. Eventually, due to normal wear and tear, accidents etc., the car will become unroadworthy and unserviceable, it is then 'scrapped' or 'wrecked' (destruction).

Prana, being the source of all matter and life must therefore similarly be involved in creation and destruction as well as protection (supporting and controlling) of the body. Iyengar confirms this when he states:

"Prana creates, protects and destroys." [63]

The Wheel Of Control (Vinaya Chakra)

Processes in the body must be controlled by various means in order to create balance. Prana, flowing through the channels and organs performs the underlying control. *Prana* then controls the elements, humors, tissues and organs in the body via the same process. This process is similar to the Wheel of Creation involving the Five Elements but by a different path, as the controlling function allows organs and humors to control others in order to retain balance.

The Wheel of Control (Vinaya Chakra) allows each element (via *Prana*) to control another element in a predetermined sequence, keeping the whole body balancing mechanisms running correctly. When this process of control fails to operate in a proper manner (in dis-ease) then those organs which are no longer under control, can erratically increase or decrease in their normal functions, causing further complications. The Wheel of Control is one of the mechanisms by which *Prana* promotes Protection, the other way is the Wheel of Support which literally 'feeds' *Prana* to every organ and tissue, in a manner to be later described in the text.

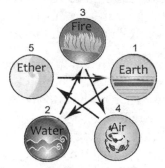

Fig.6. Cycle of Control

The clearest way of determining how this wheel (of control) functions, is to consider that control is a function opposite to the normal flow of things. The brakes (providing control) in a car although absolutely necessary, are also in opposition to what the engine/motor is trying to achieve, that is to travel forward (or backwards). In this case, the brakes attempt to counter the direction of travel (in order to provide safety). If the brakes were not operating, the car would continue to move in the same direction, rapidly gaining speed and finally crashing against another object and causing major damage/injuries, even death. So too, without this control, the body would similarly end up in a fatal situation.

As the means of control is opposite to the other functions of the body, then the Wheel of Control must similarly be in an opposite direction to creation or

63 Iyengar, BKS. (p.12).

even destruction (these two are identical). Instead of commencement in the Five Elements with Ether, the Wheel of Control starts with Earth the most physical element, and continues in the same format to reach Ether (and *Prana*). It then appears like this: Earth, Water, Fire, Wind , Ether. The previous most physical element controls the subsequent least physical one, along the line. Figure demonstrates the Wheel of Control according to the Five Elements.

Earth-Water
Earth relates to *Kapha* and in consequence Earth ensures the control of Water by providing sufficient rigidity (muscle/fat) to ensure that there is no fluid retention or looseness in the joints etc. Of course, Water also relates to *Vata* since the kidneys are also *Vata* as well as Kapha organs (via water), and in this case Earth provides the grounding and nutrients that *Vata* normally requires to prevent its catabolic effect. This has the effect of correct *Kapha* (moist) controlling *Vata* (dryness).

Water-Fire
Water normally controls Fire by increasing fluid in the body (as in water retention) and cooling down the Fire. If Water did not control the Fire (heat), then the body tissues would literally burn up. Since the kidneys deals mainly with *Vata* (by drying up the body) but also with *Kapha* by retaining fluid, then this has a similar effect to *Kapha* (cold/moist) controlling *Pitta* (heat).

Fire-Wind
Fire having a hot characteristic normally calms Wind and this is demonstrated by Fire's effect (heat) on *Vata* (coldness). One way of relaxing a *Vata* type of person is by introducing an appropriate amount of heat either internally (by diet) or by externally applying heat. Wind, having its major effect of coldness is alleviated (controlled) by heat or Fire. The use of moxibustion (*Agni*Karma) or heat therapy to a certain limit (excessive heat can over stimulate *Vata*) is therefore appropriate for a *Vata* person.

Wind -Ether
In this case, Ether represents the radiant /heat aspect of *Prana* as previously outlined.

Ether-Earth
Ether is here synonymous with *Pitta* while Earth represents *Kapha*. *Pitta* via the liver-heat controls *Kapha* as in heat controlling coldness.

PROTECTION
Elements tend to protect us from other elements that are in excess. This is also

called Control, which is a form of protection by either slowing or speeding up the action of an element.

The elements tend to protect us or control other elements in the following manner:

a. Ether protects against Earth

b. Earth protects against Water

c. Water protects against Fire

d. Fire protects against Wind

e. Wind protects against Ether

Ether Protects Against Earth

Excess Earth is restrictive, it prevents flow. Ether controls the increase of Earth by breaking it up instead of allowing it to compact and solidify. Imagine the addition of space in bread (by fermentation of yeast) which makes the bread lighter (with more spaces).

Earth Protects Against Water

Earth as an element protects us against too much Water as it helps to dry it. It slows down the flow of water which sometimes is advisable. Think of an astringent substance (e.g. pomegranate) which contains much earth, controlling the flow of diarrhea (excess water). When there are floods, sand is banked to protect properties from the excessive water flow.

Water Protects Against Fire

Water protects us from the ravages of fire. Sufficient fluids in the body prevent it from becoming too hot, so in summer (heat) we tend to drink more in order to keep cool. Water also reduces the fire and heat as for example pouring water over an open fire. Too much water though will over-control the fire and may even put it out. Movie stunt people use special liquid gel (Water) before being lit in order to protect themselves from the fire and heat.

Fire Protects Against Wind

Fire protects the body from cold wind (hot wind already has fire) which can then lead to disease by aggravating Vata or even Kapha. A Vata (Wind) person needs Fire (warmth) to protect him/herself against excess wind coldness.

Wind Protects Against Ether

Ether without Wind becomes solid (although not as solid as Earth). Earth is a more compact form of Ether. So Wind helps to move the matter (Ether and Earth) around. Ether is also combustible; it is the only element which can ignite so when in close proximity of Fire it does. As a hot type of Ether, the Wind cools it and moves it around to diffuse the heat, like an automotive radiator which diffuses the heat around, and which originates from the motor.

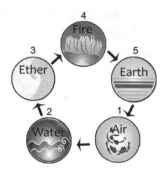

Wheel Of Support (Alamba Chakra)

The Wheel of Support relates to the method by which *Prana* supports the body, in keeping the Pranic energy flowing and by supporting each organ, tissue and element with life (*Prana*). This

Fig.7. *Cycle of Support*

is done primarily with respect to the interconnections of the elements with the humors. *Prana* traveling through *Vata*, (Wheel of Creation) must do so in all *Vata* organs conjointly. Then, likewise for the Pitta and *Kapha* organs. This wheel is not the path by which the organs' channels all connect together.

The Wheel of Support is also according to the sequence of creation but this time is according to the humors- *Vata, Pitta, Kapha*. All *Vata* organs and related elements connect together, then come all the *Pitta* organs/elements and lastly, all the *Kapha* ones.

This is demonstrated in the following table:

Humor	Element	Organs	Time
VATA	Wind-	Lung- Large Intestine	A.M.
VATA	Water(-)-	Kidney- Urinary Bladder	P.M.
PITTA	Ether-	Liver- Gallbladder	A.M.
PITTA	Fire-	Heart- Small Intestine	P.M.
KAPHA	Earth-	Spleen - Stomach	A.M.
KAPHA	Water(+)	Pericardium-Tridosha	PM.

Table. *The Element/Dosha Wheel*

The Five Elements (*pancha mahabhutas*) have been used by Ayurvedic medicine and Marmapuncture since time immemorial. It is recorded in the Vedas earlier than in any other known system of medicine. Consequently it should be used in diagnosing and treatment alongside their Doshic counterparts.

The Elements have mutual sustaining, assisting and destroying effects on each other. In so doing, they keep each other at bay and balanced. When one becomes in excess, this has an effect on another element and so on.

The Elements appear in their order of primal manifestation that is from most subtle to most physical. They are:

a. Ether

b. Wind

c. Fire

d. Water

e. Earth

The Ether element is the most subtle, it is the foundation on which the other four elements build and is the first to interface with the cosmos.

The Wind element is ether in motion creating air /wind.

The Fire element occurs by the friction created between the movement (wind) and the matter (ether). This friction creates heat which then relates to fire.

The Water element is produced by the friction or combustion of matter (ether) by the Fire which liquefies things.

The Earth element is produced by the cooling of the liquefied matter.

Creation	Dissolution	Destruction
Prana	Earth	Prana
Ether	Water	Ether
Wind	Fire	Wind
Fire	Wind	Fire
Water	Ether	Water
Earth	Prana	Earth

As a result, this process continues, especially within the body so that we are balanced; neither too hot nor too cold, not too moist nor too dry, neither too rigid nor too loose. The body's elements balance each other via the flow of Pranic energy (Prana) which is the energy of life also called the Life Force. When this energy is flowing correctly through the energetic channels called *nadis* or *dhamanis*, the Elements assist each other in a symbiotic or Parent and Child manner.

When there is a restriction of the Pranic energy, the elements begin to increase or decrease as the major control is no longer present. This increase beyond the norm for the person, results in dis-ease.

Creation of the Humors

The Ayurvedic humors (biological forces) jointly called Tridoshas (lit. 'three humors') are similarly produced from *Prana* and the Five Elements. Their appearances are exactly according to the Wheel of Creation outlined above.

There are three humors, *Vata* (Wind) which is the catabolic humor also directly dealing with the nerves, *Pitta* (Fire) which is the metabolic humor dealing with the digestive and hormonal systems and *Kapha* which is the anabolic humor relating to growth and development.

Charaka described the sequence of creation according to the Five Elements as Ether, Wind, Fire, Water and Earth respectively. This connection between them results in the creation of the three humors so that:

  (a) Ether and Wind (the first two) together create *Vata*

  (b) Fire and Water (the second group of two elements) create *Pitta*

  (c) Water and Earth (the last two) create *Kapha*.

As will be noticed each group progressively becomes more physical until reaching Earth, the most physical of the elements. Consequently, *Vata* effects are 'airy and light' in a rising direction, *Pitta* effects are medium and *Kapha* effects are heavy and in a downwards or falling direction. Chapter 4 describes this further.

Humoral Aggravation

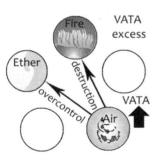

Vata Aggravation

When Vata is aggravated or in excess there is destruction of Fire and over control of Ether resulting in coldness and dryness as well as porosity (e.g. osteoporosis).

Pitta Aggravation

When Pitta is aggravated or in excess, there is over control of Air and destruction of Water resulting in dryness, fast metabolizing of tissues, nervousness, pain etc.

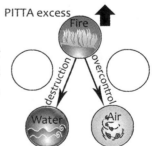

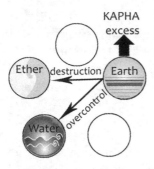

KAPHA
excess

Ether destruction Earth

overcontrol

Water

Kapha Aggravation

When Kapha is aggravated or in excess, there is over control of Water and destruction of Ether resulting in coldness, dryness and solidity (no air spaces- Ether).

The 12 Major Organs

The Twelve Organs

According to Charaka, there are various types of internal organs or viscera in the thoracic and abdominal areas. These organs (often called Kosthangas) are classified in Ayurvedic acupuncture into two types according to their structure or function.

(1) **SOLID** or Controller ORGANS

This type of organ controls the flow of energy, blood and body fluids.

These include

1. Heart (*Hridaya*) controls the flow of blood through the body, mental activity and is responsible for health of the blood vessels.

2. Lung (*Phuphusa*) controls the flow of water in the body and the flow of *Prana* or bioelectricity. It is responsible for the health of the skin and hair.

3. Liver (*Yakrit*) controls the integrity of *Prana* or bioelectricity and is responsible for the health of the tendons.

4. Spleen (*Pliha*) controls digestion and the transportation of blood. It is responsible for the muscles.

5. Kidney (*Vrikka*) controls water metabolism, is responsible for the bones and marrow and affects the reproductive organs.

6. Pericardium (*Talahridaya*) is not an organ as the others it is a membrane (*kala*) but in Ayurveda is nevertheless recognized as one due to its important physiological and energetic functions in the body. The pericardium is related to flow and therefore akin to *Kapha* (water flow humor) and the Water Element.

(2) **HOLLOW** or Storer ORGANS (also called bowels). This type of organ is responsible for the digestive, absorption and secretion processes of food and waste products. In some cases they also relate to the absorption of Pranic energy (e.g. large intestine from food).Most of these storer organs end with the suffix of *ashaya* which means: storer or container e.g. *amashaya*: container of ama, for the stomach.

These include:

1. Stomach (*Amashaya*) as with the spleen with which it is internally/externally connected, the stomach also affects digestion and the muscles.

2. Large Intestine (*Vrihdantra*) is also a site where *Prana* is absorbed into the body. Like the Lung, the large intestine has an effect on the health of the skin and hair.

3. Small Intestine (*Grahani* and also called *Laghvantra*) Just as it happens with the heart, the small intestine is necessary in the health of the blood vessels.

4. Gall Bladder (*Pittashaya*) stores bile (greenish fluid) produced by the liver and this gall or bile is used in the digestive process and is therefore also responsible for the patency of *Prana* as well as for the health of the tendons.

5. Urinary Bladder (*Mutrashaya*) is a membranous sac which stores urine after it is produced and excreted by the kidneys. It, like the kidneys affects the bones, marrow and the reproductive organs.

6. Tridosha (*Shleshmashaya*) is not an organ per se but is a generalization of the three humoral energies (VPK), their effects and functions in the human body, specifically in the torso. Tridosha is a generalization of the three areas of the trunk that represent the three humors- *Vata, Pitta* and *Kapha*.

Great attention is paid in Ayurveda to the digestive tract organs such as the Stomach, Small Intestine and Large Intestine since this is where the humors/doshas normally first accumulate and thereafter cause dis-ease by migration to other areas. The driving principle of marmapuncture, just like that of pancha-karma (five therapies) is to return the doshas back to their original sites in the g.i. tract.

Organs Interrelationships

Lung and Large Intestine (WIND)
The Lung is considered a solid organ, while the large intestine is a hollow organ.

Air (containing *Prana*) is breathed into the lungs while Prana contained in food is absorbed in the large intestine. This provides an irrefutable connection between these two organs although they are not connected together by any form of physical pipe.

Their connection is one of a functional type that is the common denominator of the element Wind (containing Prana) and as Svoboda explains:

"The health of our lungs and colon [large intestine] determines how much Prana we can absorb and how alive we feel." since.. *"We obtain Prana from our atmosphere and our food."* [64]

Frawley explains that :
"The lungs are an important site of air [wind], Vata. Here the energy of the life-force (Prana) is taken into the body." [65]

Svoboda further explains that diseases of these two organs are often interrelated and that by treating one, we often treat the other. (Svoboda, p.124).

*"**Vayu** [Wind] - Lung and large intestine."* [66]

Small Intestine and Heart (FIRE)
The small intestine has previously been described as a Fire related organ since *Agni* (fire) resides there.

These two organs have a very close relationship as the heart is considered a Fire solid organ while the small intestine (a hollow pipe) is the corresponding Fire hollow organ.

The connection between the Heart and Fire is undeniable as demonstrated by the pathological effect of Fire on an individual's heart. As Frawley explains:

"In the Ayurvedic association of Pitta (fire) with the blood, heart disease, particularly heart attacks and strokes are commonly a Pitta [fire] disorder." [67]

*"**Tejas** [Fire]- Heart and small intestine."* [68]

Kidney and Urinary Bladder (WATER)
The Kidney is related to the Bladder as both organs form the major part of the urinary system. There is a physical as well as a functional connection (via Water) between these two organs. Consequently, the Kidney is considered a

---

64 Svoboda, R., *Prakruti, Your Ayurvedic Constitution.* (p.124).
65 Frawley, D. (p.161).
66 Joshi, et al. (p.4).
67 Frawley, D. (p.171).
68 Joshi, et al. (p.4).

solid organ while the Urinary Bladder is a hollow organ (since it is not unlike a hollow sack or pipe). The connection between the Kidney and Bladder is therefore via Water. The Kidneys relate and control Bone and Marrow, both Vata tissues (dhatus). Hence this unit not only relates to Water in Kapha but also Water - (minus) in Vata.

> *"Jala* (Water- Kidney and urinary bladder (U.B.).)." [69]

Stomach / Spleen(Pancreas) (EARTH)
Earth, *Kapha*, (fat) and the Stomach are directly related to each other. The Stomach must therefore be involved not only in *Kapha* problems (e.g. fluid retention, loose joints and muscles) (Lad and Frawley, p.11). but also in the overall process of growth (muscles, fat etc.).

As Svoboda explains:

> *"all foods which increase Kapha tend to increase weight."* [70]

However, gaining weight might be done by increasing either fat or muscle content in the body, by obesity or muscle building, respectively.

> *"Prithvi (Earth- Spleen and stomach)."* [71]

Liver and Gall Bladder (ETHER)
When Ether is digested in the Liver to produce more body Ether, this element comes into close contact with the Liver fire (*BhutaAgni*) which then causes heat release. No wonder that the Liver is considered a *Pitta* (fire) organ in the body. The heat released from the Liver is mainly due to the combustion of Ether and so the Liver is a heat organ. It is then not unusual to find that diseases of a fire source (*Pitta*) (e.g. heart attacks, skin rashes) are strongest during the day when the Small Intestine and Heart's Pranic energy are strongest (11am-3pm), while the Liver and Gall Bladder reflect *Pitta* problems of a more sedate nature (hyperacidity) and emanate during the night (11pm -3 am).

> *"Akasha [Ether)- Liver and gall bladder (G.B.)."* [72]

---

69 Joshi, et al. (p.4).
70 Svoboda, *Prakruti, Your Ayurvedic Constitution.* (p.95).
71 Joshi, et al. (p.4).
72 Joshi, et al. (p.4).

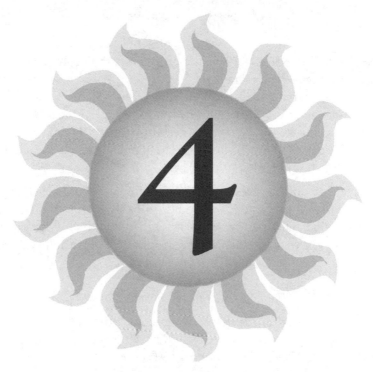

The physical and psychological manifestations of prana

Once in the body, prana transforms itself into various forces that normally maintain the body's wellbeing and that also cause different effects day by day, hour by hour. Later, prana flows through various systems of canals that themselves assist in the distribution of prana through the body. These pranic channels- also called *nadi* and *dhamani*- maintain health when they act correctly. Prana also forms inside the body various vortices of energy called *chakras*, and when prana diffuses superficially near the skin, also form lethal zones called marmas and points of treatment that are given the name of *siras*.

Tridosha

Tridosha is the 'science of the three humoral energies'. These three energies are the driving and binding forces of all the physical / psychological functions of the body. They are the nexus and core of Ayurveda, without them, it isn't Ayurveda.

The *Tridosha* is a generalization of three energies (*Vata, Pitta* and *Kapha*) which derive from *Prana* the Bio-energy / Primordial energy. *Tri* is Sanskrit for 'three', while *dosha* means a 'fault'.

While the Five Elements give the body its general qualities, the three humoral energies provide the impetus, driving or supportive force to keep it in health. Due to various causative factors, the *Tridoshas* may also lead it to dis-ease.

It is because a humoral energy is involved and is the principal source of the dis-ease (although *Prana* is the driving force of the humoral energy) that the three humoral energies are called *doshas* or 'faults'. They are also called faults because philosophically speaking humans are not perfect and hence this imperfection or fault allows us to have certain traits or characteristics that can be noticeable e.g. dry hair (*Vata* trait) . These traits together form one of three Ayurvedic constitutions (*Prakruti*) or body-types.

If the three humoral energies were perfectly in balance (*although they do have to work in harmony for health*), we would probably look totally different. It is these faults which allow us human characteristics and when unbalanced, the body will demonstrate these characteristics further in pathological changes.

States Dr. Svoboda :

"These three are forces, not substances." [73]

Thus *Vata* is made up of the first two elements: Ether and Wind, *Pitta* of the next two elements Fire and Water, while *Kapha* is made up of the last two being Water and Earth. Water is common to both *Pitta* and *Kapha*, *since water is the most abundant substance in the body.*

Meanwhile, the three humoral energies *Vata*, *Pitta* and *Kapha* normally help to bind the Five Elements together, as these three are forces not substances.

The *Tridoshas* therefore provide a mechanism for antagonistic Elements (e.g. Fire and Water) to function and exist synergistically. When these Doshas become 'faulty', the antagonism re-surfaces and disease soon follows.

Tridosha Location

The *Tridoshas* being energies are located all over the body, but there are certain sites where they are housed or where they accumulate normally. The *Tridoshas'* sites are the Primary sites where each humoral energy first accumulates or is aggravated before reflecting major symptoms.

Kapha is first aggravated in its primary site: the Stomach
Pitta is firstly aggravated in the Small Intestine: its primary site.
Vata's primary site is the Large Intestine where it is first aggravated.

From these three primary sites, the *Doshas* migrate to other sites via various means, including the blood stream. Consequently a *Kapha*-type cold may first start in the stomach and later migrates to the lungs.

---

73 Svoboda, R. *Prakruti, Your Ayurvedic Constitution.* (p.17).

Location in the Torso

Kapha- Above the breathing diaphragm is the area of *Kapha*. This is where most Kapha type problems occur-e.g. congestion, sinus problems.

Pitta- Between the diaphragm and the navel. This is where most Pitta type problems occur- e.g. Fatty liver, Cholecystitis. Abdominal distension and pain.

Vata- is located in the area below the navel. This is the area where Vata problems tend to occur, e.g. adrenal exhaustion, constipation, sciatica, elimination problems etc.

Tridoshas Qualities

- *Vata* has cold and dry attributes.

- *Pitta* has hot and moist attributes.

- *Kapha* has cold and moist attributes.

The Doshas are forces not substances, and so consequently it is the controlling action on the Elements by the *Doshas*, which produces these qualities. Dr. Frawley states:

> *"The biological humors [Vata, Pitta, and Kapha]*
> *are merely three different statuses or*
> *orientations of the life-force [Prana]."* [74]

Constitutions

Each person inherits a constitution (from the mother and father) or body-type (*prakruti*). Although each person is unique in his or her own body make-up, nevertheless, all of us fall under similar categories (body-types) which are well explained by Ayurveda.

---

74 Frawley, D. (p.108).

Vata

The combination of Ether and Wind creates the *Vata* humoral energy or *dosha*. It is:

- Catabolic
- Aggravated by cold wind.
- Nervous disposition.
- Dry.
- Protruding body joints (e.g. knees and elbows).
- Related to the period of time after middle age.

Vata Signs of Aggravation

Loss of mind / body coordination, hyperactivity of certain organs and systems leading to catabolism and decay. *Vata* almost always also involves pain.

Pitta

The combination of Fire and Water creates the *Pitta* humoral energy or *dosha*. It is:

- Metabolic.
- Aggravated by heat.
- Easily angered.
- Hot.
- Lacks body hair.
- Related to the period of time between teenage and middle age.

Pitta Signs of Aggravation

Excessive bleeding, inflammation, fever, acidity. When these affect certain body tissues they may lead to infection caused by fermentation and production of toxins, ideal food for bacteria and germs.

Kapha

The combination of Earth and Water creates the *Kapha* humoral energy or *dosha*. It is:

- Anabolic.
- Aggravated by excess cold and moisture.
- Lethargy or inactivity.

- Cold and moist.

- Excess in body hair.

- Related to the period of time from birth to teens.

Kapha Signs of Aggravation

Lethargy, phlegm, heaviness of limbs, indigestion and malabsorption of necessary nutrients.

The Tridoshas then lead towards related energies called subdoshas or dosha subtypes. These are the different manifestations in the body of Vata, Pitta and Kapha but always remembering that they are Prana in its various forms and influences. They are also consequently related to the Five Elements.

Doshic Subtypes

Just like there are five pranas which often relate to Vata, (refer to Chapter 3) (interestingly sometimes these are called e.g. *pranavata* instead of *pranavayu*), there are likewise five types of Pitta and five Kapha subtypes. They are called the doshic subtypes and are listed below:

Vata SubTypes

1. Prana Vayu

Ether-related. This is *undigested* Ether (cold and dry) not digested Ether (hot and dry), which then is later related to *Pitta*.

This subtype allows the correct **inward** action of air and of food. Principally though, it also facilitates the intake of cosmic *Prana* into the body as well as energizing and coordinating the heart, mind, our senses and consciousness. It is the welcoming party or concierge for Prana and is located in the brain and connects with the heart and chest via the throat. Consequently, normal actions like swallowing and inhaling as well as more negative actions like belching and sneezing are a reflection of this *Prana* when aggravated.

2. Udana Vayu

Wind-related (*Upward movement*). Udana Vayu is positioned in the chest and throat and facilitates normal **upward** actions such as exhaling and speech but also more negative actions such as cough, sneezing, belching and vomiting, when aggravated. It relates to our life's aspiration or upward movement in our goals. It also allows *Pranic* energy to rise or ascend. It facilitates memory when functioning correctly. When aggravated it may cause vomiting, nausea, sneezing, coughing.

3. Samana Vayu

Fire-related (*Transforming or equalizing movement*). *Samana Vayu* is located mainly in the small intestine and allows correct absorption of nutrients. It assists in **balancing** the upper portion of the torso (and body), containing major organs and its governing humor (*Kapha*), with the lower portion of the torso (and body) which contains mainly the eliminatory organs and their related governing humor (*Vata*). When aggravated, it results in indigestion and malabsorption.

4. Vyana Vayu

Water-related (*Diffusion, distribution movement*). *Vyana Vayu* governs the circulation in the body. It facilitates blood, other fluids and the nerve impulses to flow to the legs and arms. It is the **outwards** or centripetal moving *Vayu*.

5. Apana Vayu

Earth-related (*Downward movement-Stability*). *Apana Vayu* governs the downward movement of the body and is centered in the large intestine primarily and the kidney/bladder secondarily. This energy controls menstruation, urination, defecation, parturition and reproductive tissue flow. Here, the moving energy of Wind (*Vata*) and the heavy falling energy of Earth (*Kapha*) come together to produce this energy. Water absorption generally occurs in the large intestine, so that *Apana Vayu* also has a controlling interest in this activity. Correct balance of *Apana* is essential, otherwise, the body will commence to catabolize as essential ingredients will leak out via this downward action when in excess. *Apana Vayu* (outwards) being the opposite direction to *Prana Vayu* (inwards) results in these two energies controlling the other forms of *Vayu* and hence acupuncture treatment of the body normally includes needling *Prana* or *Apana's* related *marmas* or siras. Increasing earth generally results in increase of *Apana*.

Pitta Subtypes

1. Sadhaka Pitta

Ether-related. This is centered in the brain and heart and controls the subtle intellect. *Sadhaka Pitta* allows the perception of truth or reality from lies and deceptions and fantasy. Like *Tejas* in the brain, *Sadhaka Pitta* assists in metabolizing or digesting ideas. This *Pitta* has a similar movement to *Prana Vayu* as they are both Ether-related.

2. Alochaka Pitta

Wind-related. *Alochaka Pitta* is centered in the eyes and controls the ability to visually receive information. Shapes and colors will increase or decrease the humors, and these are received visually. Just like eating a heating herb, the colors or shapes of things may aggravate or sedate the humors via the eyes and finally the mind. Being Wind-related, it has an upward tendency (from eyes up to the brain) similar to *Udana Vayu*. It helps us to aspire (upwards) towards truth and knowledge.

3. Pachaka Pitta
Fire-related. *Pachaka Pitta* is located in the small intestine like *Samana Vayu* and assists circulation and the other forms of *Pitta*. It is the controller of digestion and whereas *Agni* is the digestive fire itself and also located in the Small Intestine; *Pachaka Pitta* is the energetic humor of digestion. It is related to digestive bile (gallbladder) and acid (stomach). Via the digestive process, heat is introduced into the circulation to maintain body temperature. When *Pachaka Pitta* is weak, the body may feel cooler and malabsorption may occur. When high, ulceration and indigestion may occur.

4. Bhrajaka Pitta
Water-related. *Bhrajaka Pitta* is located on the skin and controls its luster and color. It assists the absorption of vitamin D and heat through the skin, from the Sun. When vitiated, it may cause skin rashes and the discoloration of the skin. Through the absorption of heat via the skin, *Bhrajaka Pitta* assists the circulatory system and is akin to *Vyana Vayu* or the diffusing energy.

5. Ranjaka Pitta
Earth-related. *Ranjaka Pitta* found in the small intestine, liver, stomach and spleen, gives these organs' secretions their color and texture. For instance bile, blood, pancreatic juices, stools and urine. Strong coloring of these secretions may indicate derangement of its related organ. It is mainly concentrated in the blood, giving it its characteristic heat. This *Pitta* is related to *Apana Vayu* in its downward characteristics.

Kapha Subtypes

1. Tarpaka Kapha
Ether-related. *Tarpaka Kapha* is located in the brain due to its connection with subtle Ether and controls the lubrication of the brain, the heart and the nervous system. It assists in memory retention and circulation of ideas in the brain and also provides a stable basis for these ideas. It is related to *Prana Vayu* via its Ether element connection.

2. Bodhaka Kapha
Wind-related. *Bodhaka Kapha* is located (as in saliva) in the oral cavity and allows the perception of taste and assists digestion. Its aggravation, as in too much Wind affecting Water, may tend to dry this function and result in lack

of taste. Water is required for tasting. It is located in the brain also and allows maintenance of our general 'taste in good things' (e.g. clothes, activities, etc.)

3. Kledaka Kapha

Fire-related. *Kledaka Kapha* is found in the stomach and its alkaline secretions and is responsible for the first stage of digestion. It assists in liquefying the food and maintaining the correct level of water in the digestive tract. It is related to *Samana Vayu*, the balancing *Prana* in as much as it provides a balance between the digestive system and the internal body and its tissues.

4. Sleshaka Kapha

Water-related. *Sleshaka Kapha* controls the synovial fluid that is located in the body joints. As such it lubricates and allows the joints' their correct motions. It also gives them moveability. When deficient, it allows dryness of the joints as in arthritis, while in excess allows looseness and heaviness in these joints. It is related to *Vyana Vayu* via the Water element and allows correct outward movement.

5. Avalambaka Kapha

Earth-related. *Alamba* means support, thus *Alamba Chakra* or the Wheel of Support (of the Five Elements). The supporting function is mainly *Kapha*-related just like the Wheel of Destruction (catabolism) is *Vata*-related or the Wheel of Control (metabolism) is *Pitta*-related. *Avalambaka Kapha* is therefore that which supports and is primarily located in the chest area (heart and lungs). In combination with the Earth element it is related to *Apana Vayu* or downwards energy and so, if deficient may tend to allow fluids etc. to be held within (attachment to things) and cause constipation, lung congestion and obesity. It is the main energy for treatment of *Kapha* congestion.

Subdoshas treatment examples

Every one of these subtypes can be treated via acupuncture by needling its appropriate sira/marma. For instance:

Prana Vayu can be treated by using sira **Pericardium 8- P8**. This reflex point is called *Talahridaya marma* which means the Heart of the Palm *marma* and is located on the center of the palm. It is also often referred to as *Setu Manodhara Sira*, which means the Bridge point of the Pericardium. It assists in the intake and flow of *Prana* via the lungs, which it stimulates.

Vyana Vayu can be treated by using sira, **Conception 17- C17**. This is *Hridaya Marma* or the Heart point and is located in the center of the chest, halfway down the sternum. This point is also called *Vyana sira*.

Apana Vayu can be treated by the yoga sira **Spleen 6** - Sp6. This reflex point is called *Apana sira* because it is the major distal (away from the torso) point, which directly controls the action of *Apana Vayu*.

Avalambaka Kapha can be treated by using sira. **Lung 5**- L5. This is the *Kurpara Phuphusa sira* and Water element point in the Lung channel and consequently helps in clearing the lungs. It is located in the elbow crease, thumb side, anterior of elbow.

Ranjaka Pitta can be treated by using sira **Liver 2**- Lv2. This reflex point is called *Pada Kshipra marma*, *which* is located near the web of the large and first toes. It relates to the element of Fire, which it represents at this location.

Subdoshas and their siras

No.	Subdoshas	Siras
1	*Prana Vayu (Vata)*	Pericardium 8 (P8)
2	*Udana Vayu (Vata)*	Pericardium 6 (P6)
3	*Samana Vayu (Vata)*	S. Intestine 5 (SI5)
4	*VyanaVayu (Vata)*	Conception 17(C17)
5	*Apana Vayu (Vata)*	Spleen 6, UB35, C2
6	*Sadhaka Pitta*	P7, (Per8, C17)
7	*Alochaka Pitta*	Liver 3
8	*Pachaka Pitta*	Conception8, SI5
9	*Bhrajaka Pitta*	Lung 7
10	*Ranjaka Pitta*	Liver 2
11	*Tarpaka Kapha*	Pericardium 3
12	*Bhodaka Kapha*	Lung 5
13	*Kledaka Kapha*	C12, Stomach 36
14	*Sleshaka Kapha*	Kidney 10, 3D2
15	*Avalambaka Kapha*	Stomach 36, Lung 5

The reader is referred to the 700 siras section Appendix 1 for a comprehensive listing of treatment of these subdoshas by needling the appropriate sira(s).

The Tridoshic Symbol

The traditional symbol of the Tridoshas in Ayurvedic acupuncture is represented by a chakra or wheel with three spokes (supports), which demonstrate the three humors when balanced, as supporters of life. Each humor is represented by a 'tadpole' type figure. This figure consists of a circle, which contains the two elements prominent in the particular dosha (e.g. Wind and Ether for *Vata*). Each one also consists of a tail, which represents movement (like a comet tail). The tadpole is the start of life for the frog, so the elements and humors are likewise the basis of life. Consequently, there are to be found three of these 'tadpoles', one for *Vata*, one for *Pitta* and one for *Kapha*. Interestingly, the gaps between the tadpole figures actually form the spokes of the wheel. *Vata* is located at the top of the design within the Chakra circle, as it is the lightest and most subtle. *Pitta* is located on the right side (*Pitta* side of the person) and has an upward direction (like heat). *Kapha* is located on the left and has a downwards direction (like cold).

All Five Elements are consequently found in the Tridosha design, along with the three humors or doshas and the Chakra, the Pranic energy wheel. When only one humor needs to be represented by the symbol, then the other two humors are blanked (empty tadpoles) in the design, to demonstrate that although they are then in the background, they are still part of the Tridosha. The three humors are never found in isolation, all three are inter-related and necessary, in everyone.

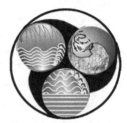

Fig. 8. *3 Doshas symbol*

Vata, *Pitta* and *Kapha* appear in the *Tridoshic* symbol in much the same way they act in the body. The *Tridoshic* symbol appears to have been used by a number of cultures but was more prevalent within the alchemical tradition of India and later Asian traditions. The center or stylized three-armed svastika, common to Indian Hinduism and Jainism is meant to represent eternality and is based on the Hindu and later Buddhist four-armed *svastika* (स्वस्तिक) which is also meant to mean a lucky or auspicious object. It also represents *dharma*. The Japanese call it mitsutomoe and is similar to the ancient Celtic *triskelion* (three-legged) design.

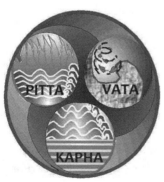

Fig. 9. *VPK symbol*

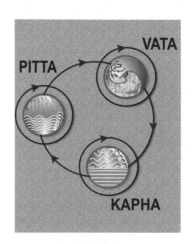

THE PHYSICAL AND PSYCHOLOGICAL MANIFESTATIONS OF PRANA

The tridosha symbol depicts Vata, Pitta and Kapha in continual circular movement and each being made up of two of the elements which themselves are in continuous motion, e.g. Wind and Ether for Vata (upper sphere), Earth and Water for Kapha (bottom sphere) and Fire and Water for Pitta (middle sphere).

Constitutional Traits

QUALITIES	VATA	PITTA	KAPHA
Complexion	darker	reddish, freckled	lighter
Dislikes	cold	heat	damp, cold
Dreams	flying, mountain chases	fire, waterfalls, fights	oceans, clouds
Eating	quickly	moderately fast	slowly
Energy level	fluctuates	moderate, high	steady
Frame	small	medium	large
Hair texture	dry, curly	straight, fine	thick, wavy
Hair color	medium/ light brown	blonde, red, early grey	dark brown, black
Hunger	fluctuating	intense, regular meals	Low
Learning	quickly, looses focus	intense focus	takes time
Learns best by	listening	visual	association
Memory	short term	overall	long term
Moods	changeable	quick-tempered	even-tempered
Others prefer the person	more settled	more tolerant	more enthusiastic
Preference of food/drinks	warm, moist, oily	cold	warm / dry
Relationships	forms friends easily	friends by values	slow but loyal
Resting pulse	Women 80-100	70-80	60-70
	Men 70-90	60-70	50-60
Sensitivity	noise	bright light	strong smells
Skin	dry	delicate	oily, smooth
Sleep	broken, light	sound, moderate	deep, long

Stress reaction	anxious, fear	irritated	calm
Self description	lively	determined	easygoing
The person speaks	quickly, excessive	clear, precise	spaced, slow
Weight	thin	average	heavy

The Trigunas

The Psychological Humors

Ayurveda believes that besides the three biological or physical humoral energies of *Vata*, *Pitta* and *Kapha*, there also exists a set of mental / psychological or higher plane 'humoral' energies which affect the thoughts and the psychological realm.

In Ayurveda, the three are often termed *Sattva*, *Rajas* and *Tamas*. They are aligned with *Sat* (pure Being), life, *Cit* (pure consciousness) light and *Ananda* (pure Bliss) love.

They may also reflect the ability (or inability) of the mind in the perception of truth. Each one of these three may 'taint' the mind in a particular direction. Tainting here does not necessarily denote a bad quality, for each one of these three qualities in the appropriate balance provides harmony.

In order for the physical body to function correctly, the mind must likewise be balanced. The *Trigunas* assist in this function.

Sattva

Sattva relates to the qualities of clarity, perception and harmony in the mind. It allows thoughts to move, akin to the action of *Prana* and *Vata*. It may provide 'enlightenment'.

Rajas

Rajas, like *Pitta* allows the digestion or development of thoughts or ideas. Anger may dominate if *Rajas* is in excess. *Rajas* is a form of *Prana* attempting to digest or form thoughts or ideas.

Tamas

Tamas relates to the humoral energy *Kapha* and allows thoughts to take shape. *Tamas*, like *Kapha* may tend towards dullness or inertia in thoughts. In excess, the person may have an inability to correctly perceive, it may lead to heaviness and inactivity and lethargy in thoughts and actions. Fear may dominate if *Tamas* is in excess. *Tamas* is a form of *Prana* but with the sole purpose of slowing down the activity of the mind that like a brake in a car, may sometimes be necessary.

A balance of all three *gunas* is important, for we may then be able to meditate, work and relax in harmony with society and Nature. Siravedhana or marma-puncture can influence these subtle principles and help to balance them by needling specific points or combination of points. Usually, points or siras along the Pericardium channel (dhamani) are used for this.

Mental Humors

Ayurveda also states that another set of terms is likewise related and similar to *Sattva*, *Rajas* and *Tamas*. These additional three are the more physical aspects of the Trigunas and can be considered their 'prodigies'. Even so, *Prana Tejas* and *Ojas* as three mental or psychological *Doshas* tend to be more widely practiced in Yoga, Ayurveda's sister science. In Ayurvedic acupuncture, both of these terminologies and descriptions are necessary as we deal with *Prana's* flow akin to Yoga, but also with *Sattva*, akin to Ayurveda.

Just as the elements allow the formation of the three biological humoral energies, so the most subtle level of the elements via the primordial energy -*Prana* allow the development of the mental humoral energies of (also called) *Prana*, *Tejas* and *Ojas*.

Prana

Sattva's functions are also akin to *Prana* (as a mental humoral energy). This mental humoral energy allows the movement of thoughts and of perception. Actually, *Prana* is believed to derive from *Sat* (pure Being). *Prana* is aligned with the element of Wind (eg movement), in its most subtle form.

Tejas

Tejas' functions are akin to Rajas and *Pitta*. Tejas means 'radiance' or glow, an aspect of Fire. *Tejas* also has the potential to digest the thoughts, emotions and ideas and give them a 'form' or shape. *Tejas* relates to the element of Fire, in its most subtle form.

Ojas

Ojas' functions are akin to *Tamas* and *Kapha*. *Ojas* is the subtle 'nutritional' energy essence, which supplies the whole of the physio-psychological organism.

Later on, *Ojas* becomes the Immune system essence, providing protection and nutrition for the entire organism (both the physical and subtle divisions). *Ojas* is also related to the element of Water, in its most subtle of forms. There are a number of siras that can be used to balance *Ojas* in the body. One of these is *Sthapani marma* or sira G24.5.

Trigunas

The *Trigunas* are therefore the concepts of *Sattva, Rajas* and *Tamas* (ultimate subtleness) aligned with *Prana, Tejas* and *Ojas* (less subtle). When treating these mental, subtle humoral energies with Marmapuncture, we are treating the *Trigunas*. As you will later see, not only does the *Tridoshas* have a *Pranic* acupuncture channel (*dhamani*) which can be used to treat imbalances of these humoral energies, but likewise so do the *Trigunas* have an acupuncture channel (*dhamani*) which can treat the higher aspects of the mind. These channels can, through their related *marmas* (or *siras*) be needled in order to produce a balance both in the biological humoral energies (*Tridoshas*) and in the subtle humoral energies (*Trigunas*).

The Tanmatras

There are five base energies or Tanmatras (lit. Primal Measure) which relate to the Five Elements but specifically with the most subtle of the sensory faculties of sight, sound, touch, smell and taste. They are the potential that allows us to smell or see but are not necessarily just vision or taste in a physical sense. They are the Five Elements prior to becoming physical objects.

The Tanmatra of:

> Sound is called *Shabda Tanmatra*
>
> Sight is called *Rupa Tanmatra*
>
> Touch is called *Sparsha Tanmatra*
>
> Taste is called *Rasa Tanmatra*
>
> Smell is called *Gandha Tanmatra*

Sense Organs (*Jnanendriyani*)

There are also five sense organs which directly relate to the Five Elements and the Tanmatras. These allow us mental experiences by providing stimuli from the outside world.

Element	Sense	Sense organ
Ether	Sound	Ear
Fire	Sight	Eye
Air	Touch	Skin
Water	Taste	Tongue
Earth	Smell	Nose

Organs of Action (*Karmendriyani*)

Each element also relates to five organs of action .For instance, Ether relates to Sound, the Ear, and also to the Mouth as we make sounds for expression and hear that expression through our ears. So too, Fire relates to Sight, and the Eyes but also relates to feet or motion.

Ether	Sound	Ear	Mouth	Expression
Fire	Sight	Eye	Feet	Motion
Air	Touch	Skin	Hands	Grasping
Water	Taste	Tongue	Uro-genital	Elimination (Urine-Semen)
Earth	Smell	Nose	Anus	Bowel Elimination

These organs therefore relate to the most subtle features of the Five Elements. These are within the subtle realm. As the elements further develop, they affect and connect with other organs which create further physical faculties and due to their connection via the different dhamanis or meridians, they further affect the physical senses. So that a particular organ such as the Liver has an effect on the Eyes. Likewise the Large Intestine has a direct effect on the Nose. The Kidneys have an effect on the Ears.

"Traditionally, the ears are described in the Ayurvedic classics as being a type of lotus, or outer flowering of the internal organs and particularly of the kidneys, which they greatly resemble in shape. Thus kidney disorders were originally the main diseases which were diagnosed by the ears." [75]

The Chakras

Chakra Channels

The Ida and Pingala are Chakra channels or subtle pranic meridians which are normally termed nadis. They have a direct relationship with the left and right 'acupuncture' or organ channels (dhamanis). The 'acupuncture' channels are those relating directly to the organs and connecting with siras. There are fourteen of these dhamanis, that is twelve organ channels and the additional mind and reproductive channels.

Ida, Pingala

The Ida deals with the *left organ channels* or *dhamanis* which deal with negative, cold, Kapha, female aspects of the body. The Pingala or Surya deals with the *right organ channels* or *dhamanis* which deal with and reflect positive, outgoing,

---

75 Wexu, M. (pp.188,189).

male, Pitta aspects of the body. A subtle imbalance of either the Ida or Pingala channels can lead to a more physical imbalance on the related organ channels according to the left or right sides of the body. The Ida and Pingala are master channels, while the organ channels are subordinate channels. Likewise the *Janma* and *Amatya dhamanis* or channels also called Artava and Shukra Nadis are subordinate channels to **Sushumna**- the master channel.

The same number of 14 channels relate to the 14 dhamanis/nadis of Marma-puncture because they are more subtle, relating to the sense organs not just the physical/organic organs. The same number appears because there is a deep relationship between the sense organs (and the channels/nadis) and the organs (and their channels/dhamanis). Ayurveda classifies the sense organs at a more subtle level than the kosthangas or physical organs.

The Sushumna is the master channel which is reflected on the outside of the body by the Conception channel (*Janma*) (*reproduction*) and on the rear of the body by the Minister channel (*Amatya*) (*brain/mind*). In Ayurvedic acupuncture it is believed that out of the Sushumna channel flow both the Janma (frontal) and Amatya (rear) channels (via prana). This happens after the Sushumna reaches the Earth chakra. Consequently, the direction of pranic flow of the Janma and Amatya channels is upwards (and linking back at the head, where Sushumna started) after the Sushumna has delivered its energy down to the root chakra.

The Chakra channels are the most subtle channels (nadis) and having an overall effect on Pranic energy and consciousness flow through the body, whereas the organ channels or dhamanis have more physical and specific effects on Pranic energy and consciousness via the organs themselves. Both channel types exist in synergy just like chakras and marmas exist in synergy. For instance the crown chakra has an external physical connection via the *Adhipati marma* (crown). The Brow Chakra has a physical counterpart in *Sthapani marma* (on middle of brow) which also connects with Minister 24.5 sira. The Palm Chakra has a counterpart in *Talahridaya marma* (palm or sole of foot) which also relates to Pericardium 8 sira.

Internally, chakra nadis connect with these chakras, and on a more physical plane, the organ channels connect with these too via their marmas or siras.

It is unfortunate that due to historical reasons the Pranic system is today only paid lip service to by some Ayurvedic practitioners who see more value or focus on physical treatment, prescribing herbs such as shatavari or ashwagandha or arjuna to balance the "Doshas" and perhaps can not see that these can also be balanced from a more subtle level via their pranic energy channels.

The Fourteen Nadis of the Chakras terminate at various apertures (sense organs) of the human body. They supply these areas with Prana and connect with the Chakras. They commence from the Sushumna and terminate at their appropriate destination carrying Prana within them. These are the most subtle types of channels, as Chakras are indeed most subtle vortices of energy/consciousness.

The Fourteen Chakra Nadis

1. *Alambusha nadi*- Root Chakra

2. *Kushu nadi*- Sex Chakra

3. *Vishvodhara nadi*- Navel Chakra

4. *Varuna nadi*- Heart Chakra

5. *Sarasvati nadi*- Throat Chakra

6. *Sushumna nadi*- Crown and Third Eye Chakras

7. *Pingala nadi*- from Third Eye to control Right side of body

8. *Ida nadi*- from Third Eye to control Left side of body

9. *Pusha nadi*- From Third Eye goes to Right Eye

10. *Gandhari nadi*- From Third Eye goes to Left Eye

11. *Payasvini nadi*- From Third Eye goes to Right Ear

12. *Shankhini nadi*- From Third Eye goes to Left Ear

13. *Yashavati nadi*- From Third Eye goes to Right Foot and Right Hand

14. *Hastijihva nadi*- From Third Eye goes to Left Foot and Left Hand

In this way, the above fourteen nadis have an overall subtle influence on the body.

The Fourteen Meridians

The 12 Dhamanis

The Twelve Dhamanis of the organs (altogether there are 24 dhamanis, 12 per left side and 12 per right side of the body) also commence from the Sushumna, infusing prana wherever they travel, connecting with their related siras (and their associated marmas) and each terminating (or commencing) at the appropriate organ. Their pranic energy flow is akin to a loop or daisy chain. Channels on the right side of the body are strongly influenced by the Pingala nadi while the channels (dhamanis) on the left side of the body are influenced by the Ida nadi.

The 2 Nadis

Artava Nadi

The Janma Nadi (*Artava nadi*) is the Conception channel and receives its energy from the Sushumna at the perineum and travels upwards at the front of the body connecting with marmas and siras along the way. When it reaches the Hridaya Marma it infuses some of its energy into the Heart itself as Hridaya Marma directly connects with the heart. From here, the Heart sends out prana through its dedicated channel (called the Heart Channel or Hridaya dhamani) away from the heart and torso to reach the end of the hand (at the little finger). Along its way, the channel connects at important sites called marmas and siras where energy circulates and interacts with the area as well as with outside of the body. This energy is then returned back to the torso via another channel which happens to connect with a hollow organ called the Small Intestine. From the Small Intestine, another channel develops, connecting with the head and traveling down the body to reach the toes (Urinary Bladder channel). Then the energy continues upwards via another channel which then connects with the organ called the Liver. So the loop of prana flows from one organ to the next, according to this process.

The energy through the organs and their channels therefore form a loop. The flow through the Amatya and Janma nadis therefore fall outside of this loop, as a separate system, a separate loop. Once the energy is returned back to the Heart, it travels to Hridaya Marma and continues its journey upwards along the Janma Nadi to reach the mouth where it terminates and infuses back into the Sushumna.

Shukra Nadi

The Amatya Nadi (*Shukra nadi*) is the Minister channel which also commences at the perineum traveling upwards along the back of the body it reaches the mouth also while traveling along the back and top of the head, forehead, nose and top lip. Along this channel are a number of important marmas such as *krikatika, simanta, adhipati, sthapani* etc and their related siras.

The fourteen dhamanis therefore have a more physical or even specific effect on the body. They can influence very specific areas of the body, including the physical emotional and psychological states, via their unique individual acupoints or siras, something that is difficult to do via the Chakra nadis. In fact, when we treat the chakras with gems, massage etc, we are in essence treating the related sira, which affects the associated marma which then has an effect on the chakra.

Chakras

Chakras are subtle vortices of energy aligned with the central Sushumna nadi. Chakras are not physical locations but are instead located in the subtle body. They are directly related to various marmas which are like external gates to the chakras. Each chakra relates to a specific marma which is a zone on a more physical plane.

Chakras relate to the Five Elements and to Prana and they are located down the body in the same form of development as the Five Elements.

Hence:

The first chakra (*Sahasrara*) relates to Prana in its most subtle form, that is the highest psychological form.

The second (*Ajna*) also relates to Prana and its mind, perception connection.

The third (*Vishuddha*) relates to Ether.

The fourth (*Anahata*) relates to Wind.

The fifth (*Manipura*) relates to Fire.

The sixth (*Svadhishthana*) relates to Water.

The seventh chakra (*Muladhara*) is the Earth Chakra which is development into its most physical form.

Chakra	Element	Related Marma	Related Sira
Crown Chakra	Prana	Adhipati Marma	Governing 20
Brow Chakra	Prana	Sthapani Marma	G 24.5, G16
Throat Chakra	Ether	Nila, Manya	Stomach 9, Large Intestine 18, C23, G14
Heart Chakra	Wind	Hridaya Marma	C17, G10
Navel Chakra	Fire	Nabhi Marma	Conception 8, G6
Sex Chakra	Water	Kukundara, Vitapa	GB29, K11, C6, G3
Root Chakra	Earth	Guda Marma	Governing 1, Conception 1

There are some who number the chakras differently, with Sahasrara as 7th Chakra and the *Muladhara* Root Chakra as first. This does not change their names, or their locations or attributes in any way. The above description and numbering is based on pranic flow which occurs first at the sahasrara and descends to finally reach the root chakra (7th).[76]

Pranic flow therefore travels downwards first along the Sushumna nadi, inte-

---

76 Dr. David Frawley. *Ayurveda And The Mind.* Lotus, USA p.146.

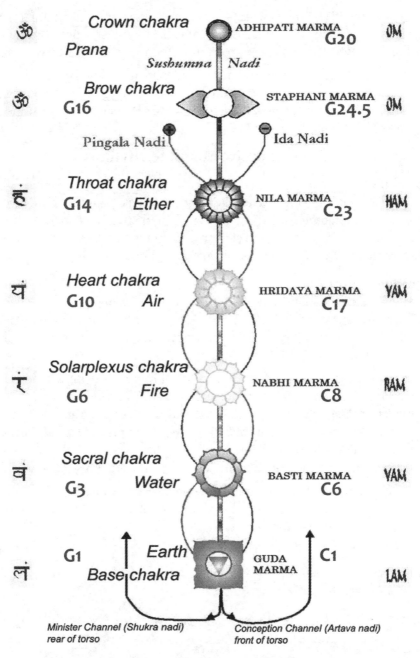

Chakras, Marmas & Related Siras

Fig. 10. Chakras, nadis, their marmas and their siras

grates with the Ida (-) and Pingala (+) nadis and other subtle nadis, then travels upwards along the Shukra and Artava nadis before infusing itself through the 24 dhamanis which then allow prana's return to the Sushumna nadi once again.

It is also believed that Prana also enters and exits the body through the siras/marmas in much the same way an airport is a gateway that allows entry and exit into a city or country. Hence marmapuncture facilitates this entry and exit of prana through the skin.

Ayurvedic circadian bio-rhythms

Mandala

The *Pranic Mandala* or Ayurvedic Bio-Rhythm Clock is a very helpful tool in order to understand how diseases are aggravated at various times of the day, which humor, related organ, and element are aggravated as well as deciphering which organ-needling channel is affected and should be utilized.

Mandala- *definition*

The word *mandala* originates from the Sanskrit *manda*, which means 'essence', and *la*, which stands for 'seizing' or 'enclosing' [77]. Its full import means a device which assists in grasping (seizing) the knowledge (essence or prana) of the Ayurvedic biorhythms of Ayurvedic acupuncture. A container of the essence.

The Pranic Mandala represents the *Pranic* flow through the body in its actual and disguised forms (e.g. elementary, doshic, etc.) and is divided into six humoral segments representing the three doshas, repeated twice within any 24-hour day/night. Each segment is itself divided into two related organ sections. Likewise, each segment is related to one of the Five Elements. As well, the appropriate *Pranic* channels are easily identifiable within each humoral segment.

The *mandala* petals, twelve in number represent the *Pranic* flow through the twelve major organs/channels and the division of a 24-hour day into twelve sections, each of two hours duration.

Doshic Times

Professor Dr. Ranade (ex Ayurvedic Dean, Poona University) states the dosha times very clearly:

"Movement of the Doshas Through The Cycle Of Time

Kapha	Pitta	Vata	
Day	7am-11am	11am-3pm	3pm- 7pm
Night	7pm-11pm	11pm-3am	3am-7am ." [78]

77 Ferdinand D. Lessing, Alex Wayman. *Introduction To The Buddhist Tantric Systems*. Motilal Banarsidass, India 1978. Volume 20. (p. 270).
78 Ranade, A. *Natural Healing Through Ayurveda*. (p.43).

Vata Times

Vata is normally considered to be aggravated daily in the early morning and in the afternoon. Each one of these two time sequences, although relating to *Vata*, demonstrate different types of *Vata* symptoms. This occurs due to the *Vata* type of organs (primary organs) (Lungs/Large Intestine) which can be affected in the morning and the different *Vata* ones (secondary organs) (Urinary Bladder/Kidney) affected in the afternoon, according to an energy cycle.

Charaka deciphers the *Vata* time in the *Nidansthana* chapter by stating *Vata* (as in a *Vata*-type fever) has its

> *"Occurrence or aggravation in the afternoon [or] during dawn."* [79]

Pitta Times

Pitta is aggravated during the day at the time of most heat (after 12 noon). This is according to the Sun (e.g. a sundial). *Pitta* therefore can reflect its morbidity effects for four hours, from just before noon (11 a.m.) till the afternoon (Heart/Small Intestine), that is before 3 p.m. and at night between 11pm and 3am. Charaka once again states in the *Nidansthana* that *Pitta* has:

> *"simultaneous manifestation or aggravation in the entire body during the mid-day [and] mid-night ..."* [80]

Kapha Times

Kapha times occur before noon and before midnight, after *Vata's* aggravation time in the morning and in the evening. Kapha therefore reflects its effects between 7am-11am and between 7pm-11pm. Charaka (in *Nidansthana*) states that *Kapha* (type fever) can demonstrate:

> *"simultaneous manifestation or aggravation in the entire body during the fore-noon [and] in the evening."* [81]

Primary and Secondary Organs

Each humor or dosha has two primary organs (both a solid and a hollow type) and two secondary organs (a solid and a hollow type). The primary organs appear to have a direct connection with the appropriate humor- e.g. the Large Intestine with Vata, Small intestine with Pitta and the Stomach with Kapha.

The secondary organs have an indirect but real connection with the humor- e.g. Kidney with Vata.

---

79 Sharma R. and Dash, B. (p.24).
80 Ibid. (p.22).
81 Sharma R. and Dash, B. (p.24).

Humor	Primary organs	Secondary organs
Vata	Lung/ *Large Intestine*	Kidney/ Urinary Bladder
Kapha	Spleen/ *Stomach*	Pericardium/ Tridosha
Pitta	Heart/ *Small Intestine*	Liver/ Gallbladder

Organ Pranic Sequences

As explained above, each organ has an individual two-hour duration during which *Prana* is at its most flourishing. After these two hours, another one of the twelve organs receives the energy and itself becomes the most flourishing for a length of two hours. This process continues in a daisy-chain format until the twenty-four hours of the day have been exhausted and a new day begins.

The method by which to determine which organ appears at what time can best be understood by following this simple rule:

a) Within the same humor only dissimilar types of organs can connect together (hollow and solid).

b) Between different humors only similar types of organs can sequentially connect together (solid-solid or hollow-hollow).

It must therefore be concluded that for a period of four hours, each humor can be aggravated, twice in a day. This is because during those times, the humors' interrelated organs each have an abundance of Pranic energy. Each organ retains this abundance or peak of energy during two hours, after which, it hands the energy peak to the next organ in line, via this new organ's Pranic channel (Nadi/dhamani).

Appropriate Times for Food

Ayurveda recommends, in accordance with the mandala that only *Vata* and *Pitta* people should partake in breakfast approximately at the time of sunrise (before *Kapha* time). *Kapha* people should ideally skip breakfast.

Lunch should be eaten at approximately after 11 am so that its effect can appropriately occur by noon (*Pitta* time). Likewise, evening meal time should be eaten before sunset so that its effect does not occur well into the *Pitta* time (11pm-3am) and thus allow a restful sleep which is not in unison with the digestion of the food.

Treatment According to Mandala Time

In order to treat a particular problem, which may be aligned to the appropriate time of day or night, we need to first establish whether the organ involved has an excess or deficiency of Pranic energy.

After having established this by various diagnostic means, we may then commence its treatment.

The Pranic energy commences to rise at odd hours, reaching a peak at even hours and then declining once again to allow the next organ/channel to reach a peak. For instance, an asthma syndrome may occur at *Vata* time (3am-7am) and may affect the Lung (3-5am). The peak of energy in the Lung and its channel occurs at 4 am.

Treatment of an **excess** of Pranic energy is carried out *after* or *at* the peak of *Prana*.

Treatment of a **deficiency** of energy is carried out *before* the peak of Pranic energy in the organ/channel.

Diagonal Effects of the Humors

According to the *Mandala*, the two diagonally-opposite humors relate to the same humoral energy, but twelve hours apart. Consequently, *Vata* can be highlighted twice in one day, the *primary Vata* between 3am-7am and the *secondary Vata* between 3pm and 7pm. each one being diagonally opposite.

Pitta is likewise represented between 11am-3pm (primary *Pitta*) and 11pm and 3am (secondary *Pitta*). Kapha appears between 7am-11am (primary *Kapha*) and 7pm-11-pm (secondary *Kapha*), its diagonally opposite partner.

As *Prana* increases to a peak at the appropriate time in an organ/channel, so its diagonally opposite counterpart is required to donate some of its own *Prana* to accommodate the peak. This does not result in a total drain of *Prana* but only in a lessening of the amount contained in the organ/channel.

Where there currently exists an imbalance in this humor, the lessened amount of *Prana* in the organ/channel now means that *Prana* looses its control over it and the organ reacts negatively, erratically.

To take an example, a person suffering from a *Vata* imbalance may wake up a number of times between 3am-7am (primary) and may need to evacuate the bladder, as the kidney /bladder can no longer control and retain the urine. However, this time is actually the Lung and Large intestine time (3am-7am). Insomnia of this type is due to *Vata*, occurring at the primary time (lung/large intestine) but via a diagonally opposite *Vata* secondary effect (kidney/bladder).

Likewise, during the secondary *Vata* time (3pm-7pm) the person may suffer from lethargy. This will occur because the diagonally opposite organs of the primary *Vata*, the Lung and the Large Intestine, have a lessened amount of *Prana*, which is taken by the secondary *Vata* organs of the Kidney and Bladder and so consequently, not enough oxygen / *Prana* can enter the lungs/large intestine unit to be absorbed into the body. Lack of oxygen (and *Prana*) to the cells will result in tiredness/lethargy.

Similar effects occur to the other two humoral energies, *Pitta* and *Kapha* in a diagonally opposite fashion.

Seasonal Influences

According to Ayurveda, the seasons of the year have an influence on the humoral energies and consequently the health of the person.

In India, seasons are classified under six headings. These seasons are directly related to the six humoral effects of the *Pranic Mandala*.

There is Autumn, Summer, Winter and Spring, however these are also divided into Late Winter, Early Winter, Late Spring and Early Spring.

As a consequence the six seasons are as follows:

- Autumn
- Early Winter
- Late Winter
- Early Spring
- Late Spring
- Summer

Autumn -	increases *Vata* (Wind)
Early Winter -	increases *Vata* (Water-)
Late Winter -	increases *Kapha* (Earth)
Early Spring -	increases *Kapha* (Water+)
Late Spring -	increases *Pitta* (Ether)
Summer -	increases *Pitta* (Fire)

The seasons affect the Doshas as above.

Consequently, *Kapha* is increased during the seasons of Late Winter (*Earth*) and Early Spring (*Water*+), due to these elements' qualities of cold (*Earth*) and dampness (Water +) [82].

Vata is increased during the seasons of Autumn (*Wind*) and Early Winter (*Water*-) due to these elements' qualities of cold (Wind) and dryness (Water -) (Ranade, p.43). In some cases, Wind is also drying in effect.

Similarly, *Pitta* is increased during Late Spring (*Ether*) and Summer (*Fire*), due to these elements' qualities of heat (Ranade, p.43).

A person of a particular constitution (*Vata* Prakruti) needs to be aware to avoid increasing its related humoral energy (*Vata dosha*) especially during the seasons of Autumn and Early Winter, when these can become totally deranged and cause diseases or imbalances of the organism.

---

82 Ranade, (p.43).

A diet that would suit the person must take these increases into account, in order to balance or reduce the related dosha instead of increasing it during a particular season.

In the *Pranic Mandala,* these seasons are clearly shown alongside their related humoral energies.

Directional Influences

The Earth spins on its axis and it has a magnetic North and South Pole. Although both poles are extremely cold, this has nothing to do with their magnetic effects on objects and living things.

The North Pole causes a stimulating effect on the organism, which by its very action creates friction (through movement), this is then translated as heat. So the North Pole relates to *Pitta* and Fire.

The South Pole on the other hand has a slowing effect, causing coldness. This is related as a general rule to *Kapha* and *Vata.*

Northerly direction
With regards to direction, traveling often in a northerly direction can cause heat and inflammation.

Southerly direction
Traveling South can cause coldness and stagnation (the kidneys and bladder may decrease its normal function and as a consequence fluid may be retained within the body- e.g. in the ankles).

Westerly direction
When traveling West, the effect is of a *Vata* (Wind) increase as this is contrary to the spinning of the planet, which travels towards the East but with the on-coming Wind (and *Prana*) (from the East, just like the Sun).

Easterly direction
When traveling East, this is along the planet's direction but against the oncoming Wind, which then causes friction and heat, thereby related to *Pitta* (Ether). This *Pitta* is less hot than the North *Pitta.*

Centrifugal direction
Kapha (Water +) causes a directional movement *away from the center,* to diffuse to all parts of the body. The centrifugal direction therefore is related to *Kapha,* Water+, and Early Spring which itself stimulates this centrifugal direction.

Centripetal direction

Kapha (Earth) is also involved in a directional movement *towards the center,* due to Earth's cold, astringent qualities.

Increasing *Kapha*, might either have a centrifugal direction or else a centripetal direction, dependent on the element involved.

Channels' Pranic Flow

The channels' direction of flow of Pranic energy follows exactly that depicted in the *Mandala*. The sequence does not change. Each channel connects with its previous one in a permanent manner. For instance the Lung channel connects with the Large Intestine channel, then this channel with the Stomach channel, which then connects with the Spleen channel etc. according to the Pranic flow through them.

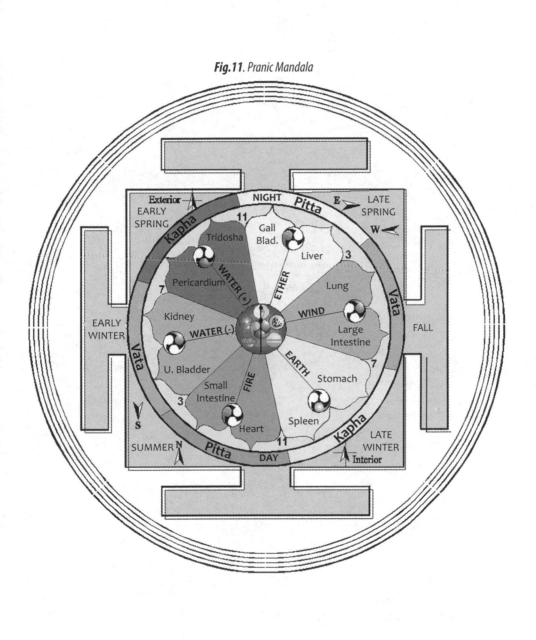

Fig. 11. Pranic Mandala

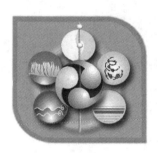

Ayurvedic acupuncture channels in the body

The Pranic channels

According to Indian traditional sources there are literally thousands of channels or meridians in the body, connecting with every living structure, that is each cell, tissue, organ and system. Some of these channels are related to visible substances, like the urinary and digestive systems channels (srotas), others connect with the subtle flow of energy (dhamanis and nadis).

Lad and Frawley explain that Ayurveda understands the body as consisting of an undeterminable number of channels [83] and that some of these channels can be aligned with the Western understanding of human physiology while others are closely aligned with the Oriental concepts of meridians. Health is maintained by providing a proper balance in the flow of prana or life force within these meridians or channels [84].

The acupuncture channels are those channels which carry *Prana* or Life energy throughout the body but which also connect with a number of areas on the body surface which can be pierced to create a balance effect on the channel.

---

83 Lad & Frawley. (p.18).
84 Ibid. (p.20).

There are other channels also such as the ones connecting with the Ayurvedic and Yoga Chakras or energy flywheels.

Sushruta explains that channels carry the subtle rasa, which we also call Prana. *Dhamani* is the channel that carries prana to and from the 12 human organs while *Nadis* relate to the Conceptual channels (Artava & Shukra Nadis) and to chakras and sense organs. Conceptual because they both relate to the brain (concept) and the reproductive organs (conception). Irrespective of what names we call these channels, they still carry prana along the body and eventually reach marmas and siras (acupoints).

Dhamanis

Sushruta also explains that the 24 organ channels (dhamanis) (belonging to the 12 organs) are classified according to their direction of pranic flow. Although, some of the organs have ascending or descending functions or both, we refer to these flow directions in this book according to the flow direction of the organ channels, not the organs themselves. There are ten which have ascending nature (*dhatu dhamanis*), ten with descending nature (*ashaya dhamanis*) and four which are termed as transverse or (*tiryag dhamanis*) (Joshi et al p.4).

Each of the twelve organs mentioned above have dual channels, that is, one along the right side of the body and one along the left side of the body. Hence there are literally 24 of these channels or dhamanis or two sets of 12 channels.

"These channels are described [by Sushruta] under five Mahabhutas namely:

- *Akasha - (Ether) Liver and gall-bladder*
- *Vayu –(Air) Lung and large intestine*
- *Teja- (Fire) Heart and small intestine*
- *Jala- (Water) Kidney and urinary bladder*
- *Prithvi- (Earth) Spleen and stomach."* [85]

"According to Sushruta there are twenty four Dhamanis as shown below:

- *10 Ascending Dhamani*
- *10 Descending Dhamani*
- *4 Transverse Dhamani. "* [86]

---

85 Drs. B.K.Joshi, R.L.Shah, G.Joshi. (p.4).
86 Ibid. (p.4).

By descending flow, we mean that the pranic energy through the meridians travels away from the organ(s) and downwards along the arm or leg. Conversely, by ascending flow we mean that the pranic energy flows towards the organ(s) upwards along the arm or leg.

Nevertheless, some organs have ascending nature and some have descending nature in their functions (not pranic flow). For instance, the lung has both ascending (exhaling) and descending (inhaling). The large intestine has a descending nature (elimination) as has the urinary bladder.

Figure 12. Organs' pranic energy flow directions

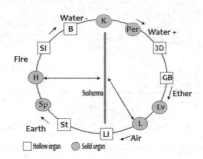

The Descending channels have pranic energy which always travels away from the torso along the limbs, while the ascending channels have pranic energy which always travels towards the torso, along the limbs.

The Transverse of *tiryag* channels do not relate to organs per se, they are connected to the concept of pericardium and tridosha. Hence they are described as transverse, their effects transverse the torso.

Descending Channel	Ascending Channel	Transverse Channel
Ashaya dhamani	*Dhatu dhamani*	*Tiryag dhamani*
1. Lung	11. Large Intestine	21. Pericardium
Left Side channel	*Left Side channel*	*Left Side channel*
2. Lung	12. Large Intestine	22.Pericardium
Right Side channel	*Right Side channel*	*Right Side channel*
3. Heart	13. Small Intestine	23.Tridosha/Shleshmashaya
Left Side channel	*Left Side channel*	*Left Side channel*
4. Heart	14. Small Intestine	24. Tridosha/Shleshmashaya
Right Side channel	*Right Side channel*	*Right Side channel*

5. Stomach *Left Side channel*	15. Spleen *Left Side channel*	
6. Stomach *Right Side channel*	16. Spleen *Right Side channel*	
7. Urinary Bladder *Left Side channel*	17. Kidney *Left Side channel*	
8. Urinary Bladder *Right Side channel*	18. Kidney *Right Side channel*	
9. Gall Bladder *Left Side channel*	19. Liver *Left Side channel*	
10. Gall Bladder *Right Side channel*	20. Liver *Right Side channel*	

It is via the dhamanis or pranic meridians that Vata, Pitta and Kapha exists in the extremities since they interact between themselves to allow the doshas' flow.

It is through the common connection of a channel with its related channel- *related by the same Element* that allows this to occur. For instance, it is through the Heart and Small Intestine channels and their common relationship with the element of Fire which allows Pitta to exist and flow through the arms.

Vata Dhamanis in the Arm

The arm has two Pranic channels that relate to *Vata*, and they are the Large Intestine and the Lung. Each arm has one set of these two channels.

Lung (*Phuphusa*)

Channel Name: Phuphusa Dhamani

Channel Energy Flow: Descending flow

Mandala Energy Time: 3 am-5 am

Lung Channel Syndromes: Demonstrates and can treat syndromes typical of lung and respiratory system disorders. Via *Vata* and Wind it has an effect on the skin, and can also treat disorders of its related organ - the Large Intestine.

Number of Siras: 11 siras

Sira Numbering System: No. 1 commences at organ, number 11 concludes at thumb.

Large Intestine (*Sthulantra/Vrihdantra*)

Channel Name: Vrihdantra Dhamani

Channel Energy Flow: Ascending flow

Mandala Energy Time: 5 am-7 am

Large Intestine Channel Syndromes: The Large Intestine channel can exhibit syndromes akin to the Lung channel, however it also treats disorders associated with pain, disorders located along the trajectory of the channel and can be used for surgery analgesia of the throat, specifically of the thyroid gland.

Number of Siras: 20 siras

Sira Numbering System: No. 1 commences at index finger, number 20 concludes at side of nostril.

Kapha Dhamanis in the Arm

The arm has two Pranic channels which relate to *Kapha*, and they are the Pericardium and the *Tridosha* (3D). Each arm has one set of these two channels.

These two organs have their arm channels connecting with each other and *Prana* flows along one and then the other.

Tridosha (3D) (*Shleshmashay*)

Channel Name: Shleshmashay Dhamani

Channel Energy Flow: Ascending flow

Mandala Energy Time: 9 pm-11 pm

Tridosha Channel Syndromes: The *Tridosha* channel can treat exhibiting syndromes such as blockages- e.g. constipation, nerve paralysis, and also pain especially along the channel trajectory- the arm. It has a major effect on the ear, which the channel physically surrounds around its perimeter.

Number of Siras: 23 siras.

Sira Numbering System: No. 1 commences at ring finger, number 23 concludes at outside end of eyebrow.

Pericardium (*Manodhara/Talahridaya*)

Channel Name: Talahridaya Dhamani

Channel Energy Flow: Descending flow

Mandala Energy Time: 7 pm-9 pm

Pericardium Channel Syndromes: The Pericardium channel can treat exhibiting syndromes such as schizophrenia, manic depression, nervousness, palpitation, anxiety and erratic heartbeat. It can also treat some heart diseases (e.g. angina) and disorders of the arm, where the channel is located.

Number of Siras: 9 siras.

Sira Numbering System: No. 1 commences at organ, number 9 concludes at the middle finger.

Pitta Dhamanis in the Arm

The arm has two Pranic channels that relate to *Pitta*, and they are the Heart and the Small Intestine channels. Each arm has one set of these two channels. These two organs have their arm channels connecting with each other and *Prana* flows along one and then the other.

Heart (*Hridaya*)

Channel Name: Hridaya Dhamani

Channel Energy Flow: Descending flow

Mandala Energy Time: 11am-1 pm

Heart Channel Syndromes: The Heart channel can treat exhibiting syndromes such as heart disease, Pitta problems (e.g. sweating) some nervous disorders mainly dealing with the brain and the heart (as the Pericardium) as well as disorders of the areas which the channel traverses- arm.

Number of Siras: 9 siras.

Sira Numbering System: No. 1 commences at the chest (near axilla), number 9 concludes at inner corner of nail of the little finger.

Small Intestine (*Grahani/Laghvantra*)

Channel Name: Laghvantra Dhamani

Channel Energy Flow: Ascending flow

Mandala Energy Time: 1 pm- 3 pm

Small Intestine Channel Syndromes: The Small Intestine channel can treat syndromes :

a) of the small intestine organ proper

b) and those relating to heat or inflammation especially along the trajectory of the channel as earlier described.

Number of Siras: 19 siras.

Sira Numbering System: No. 1 commences at outside corner of nail of little finger and number 19 concludes near the tragus of the ear.

Vata Dhamanis in the Leg

The leg too, has two Pranic channels that relate to *Vata*, and they are the Kidney and Urinary Bladder channels. Like the arm, each leg has one set of these two channels. The Urinary Bladder is a site of *Vata* according to Charaka. Both of these are *Vata* secondary organs having a direct effect on *Vata* via the kidney/ bladder drying action on the body.

Kidney (*Vrikka*)

Channel Name: Vrikka Dhamani

Channel Energy Flow: Ascending flow

Mandala Energy Time: 5 pm-7 pm

Kidney Channel Syndromes: The Kidney channel will often demonstrate syndromes such as those relating to

a) the reproductive system,

b) the urinary system and adrenals (affected by stress)

c) bone (*Vata*) imbalances and fluid retention

d) as a *Vata* organ it also affects the nerves (bone marrow).

Number of Siras: 27 siras.

Sira Numbering System: No. 1 commences at the sole of the foot, number 27 concludes at the upper section of the thorax

Urinary Bladder (*Mutrashaya*)

Channel Name: Mutrashaya Dhamani

Channel Energy Flow: Descending flow

Mandala Energy Time: 3 pm-5 pm

Urinary Bladder Channel Syndromes: The Urinary Bladder reflects syndromes akin to those of the kidneys especially lethargy, lower back pain and disorders of the urinary system and reproductive system especially during its peak time of 3-5 pm. It can also treat pain and problems located on the locality of the Bladder channel's trajectory along the body.

Number of Siras: 67 siras.

Sira Numbering System: No. 1 commences at inside corner of eye, number 67 concludes at the side of the little toe nail.

Kapha Dhamanis in the Leg

The leg has two Pranic channels that relate to *Kapha*, and they are the Spleen and Stomach. Each leg has one set of these two channels.

These two organs have their leg channels connecting with each other and *Prana* flows along one and then the other.

Spleen (*Pliha*)

Channel Name: Pliha Dhamani

Channel Energy Flow: Ascending flow

Mandala Energy Time: 9 am-11 am

Spleen Channel Syndromes: The Spleen channel demonstrates syndromes such as

a) those relating to the digestive, metabolic and immune mechanisms

b) muscle tissue (and soft tissue including skin) disorders

c) of areas which the channel crosses.

Number of Siras: 21 siras.

Sira Numbering System: No. 1 commences at inner corner of the big toe nail and number 21 concludes at the side of the body, underneath the axilla (armpit area).

Stomach (*Amashaya*)

Channel Name: Amashaya Dhamani

Channel Energy Flow: Descending flow

Mandala Energy Time: 7 am -9 am

Stomach Channel Syndromes: The Stomach channel demonstrates syndromes such as:

a) disorders of the stomach and its related spleen/pancreas

b) blockage type imbalances in the abdominal organs and reproductive organs (via its related Spleen channel)

c) disorders affecting the areas where the channel traverses.

Number of Siras: 45 siras.

Sira Numbering System: No. 1 commences underneath the middle of the lower eyelid, number 45 concludes at the second toe.

Pitta Dhamanis in the Leg

There are two Pranic channels in the leg which relate to *Pitta*, these being the Liver and Gall bladder channels. There is one set of these two channels in each leg.

Liver (*Yakrt*)

Channel Name: Yakrt Dhamani

Channel Energy Flow: Ascending flow

Mandala Energy Time: 1 am-3 am

Liver Channel Syndromes: The Liver channel can treat exhibiting syndromes such as

a) disorders of the Liver organ proper

b) pain relief, e.g. headaches etc. The Kurccha *marma* (Lv.3) in the foot is a direct relative to the Kurccha *marma* in the hand (LI 4), both of which are major analgesic points of the body and share the same traditional name

c) muscle and soft tissue disorders of the leg.

d) reproductive system disorders (where the channel traverses), especially those dealing with hemorrhaging.

Number of Siras: 14 siras.

Sira Numbering System: No. 1 commences at the big toe, number 14 concludes just below the diaphragm on the front of the body

Gall Bladder (*Pittashaya*)

Channel Name: Pittashaya Dhamani

Channel Energy Flow: Descending flow

Mandala Energy Time: 11pm- 1am

Gall Bladder Channel Syndromes

The Gall Bladder channel can treat syndromes

a) of the Gall Bladder organ proper and of the Liver.

b) and those relating to heat or inflammation especially along the trajectory of the channel as earlier described (including eye, ear and neck)

c) as well as pain and paralysis in the leg where the channel traverses.

Number of Siras: 44 siras.

Sira Numbering System: No. 1 commences at the outside corner of the eye, while number 44 concludes at the corner of the nail of the fourth toe.

The Thirteenth and Fourteenth Nadis

Just as there are fourteen *Srotas* in Ayurveda, (although there are two additionally exclusive ones for the female), so too there are fourteen *nadis* or dhamanis (channels) in Marmapuncture. The additional two comprise of what are called the Conception or Birth channel, in *Sanskrit*: **Janma Nadi** (and also Artava Nadi) and the Minister channel called **Amatya Nadi** (Also called Shukra Nadi)

These two channels relate to the Ayurvedic concept of the two *Extraordinary* organs- mainly the **brain** (under *Amatya Nadi*) and the **reproductive organ** (under *Janma Nadi*) (the Conceptual channels). These two channels are related to the *Sushumna Nadi* or yogic channel located along the center of the spine and communicating with the major chakras or energy vortexes.

Conception Channel

Channel Name: Janma Nadi and Artava Nadi.

Channel Energy Flow: Ascending flow

Conception Channel Syndromes: The Conception channel will often demonstrate syndromes such as those relating to

a) the reproductive system,

b) urinary system

c) breasts and lactation (the channel pranically connects the uterus with the breasts)

d) heart and lung disorders (C17 is the *Hridaya Marma* or heart *marma*- also relating to the pericardium organ proper).

e) Pain sensitivity along most of the Conception channel, between the groin and breasts may often indicate either:

i) a major reproductive disorder

ii) or else the possibility of pregnancy.

Number of Siras: 24 siras. Including 5 Chakras/Marmas

Sira Numbering System: No. 1 commences at the perineum, number 24 concludes at the center, directly below the bottom lip.

Minister Channel

Channel Name: Amatya Nadi and Shukra Nadi

Channel Energy Flow: Ascending flow

Minister Channel Syndromes: The Minister channel reflects syndromes relating to dysfunctions in nerves, immunity as well as brain function. This is why G20 or Amatya 20 (*Adhipati marma*) (affects pineal function) is the best mind and body relaxing *marma* as well as the best psychological and neurological treatment *marma*, while G15 (*Krikatika marma*) is the most powerful body immune stimulant point. G 24.5 halfway between the eyebrows is called *Sthapani marma*, is also the Brow Chakra of Yoga and regulates pituitary function necessary for correct hormonal conduction. Such is the importance of the Minister channel.

Number of Siras: 28 siras.

Sira Numbering System: No. 1 commences near rectum, number 28 concludes at the middle of the top gum.

Srotas

The word *Srotas* derives from the Sanskrit word *sru* which means 'flow'. It is therefore a channel or conduit which allows the flow of things through the body. These things may be blood, plasma, urine, feces, and so on.

Ayurveda understands the body as consisting of innumerable channels or srotas which basically supply the different types of tissues in the body. This can be likened to a system of canals which serve to supply nourishment to the organs and tissues of the body. By correct flow, they also facilitate cleaningness (removal of wastes).

When these channels allow excessive flow, the tissues become flooded and functions become hyperactive. When the channels restrict flow (deficient) this results in congestion of wastes and possible drying up of the tissues.

When any of the humors (*doshas*) are in excess, this may cause them to move into the channels and cause flow in the wrong direction.

"Maintaining the proper flow in the channels is essential to health and to the prevention of disease. Some of these systems [channels] are identical to the system

of western physiology; others are similar to the meridian concept of Chinese medicine." [87]

Iyengar mentions that:

*"The Shiva Samhita mentions 350,000 nadis of which **fourteen** are stated to be important."* [88]

Generally though, the physiological channels are called srotas while the energetic channels are called *nadis* and *dhamanis*.

Channels can be blocked by food which has a heavy nature (*Kapha* and *Ama* [89] increasing). In order to clear these channels, a lighter type diet should be attempted and therapy which promotes flow of *Prana* should be carried out. These include acupuncture, *marma* massage, *Pranayama*, meditation, yoga and so forth.

Srotas description

There are principally 14 major *Srotas* or channels in the body (the female has sixteen while the male has only 14, however the additional two channels of the female could rightly come under the auspices of the reproductive channels thus forming 14 srotas), just like there are 14 organ needling meridians (including Artava nadi and Shukra nadi) and there are 14 chakra nadis.

These srotas are divided into 5 distinct groups of channels.

The first group connects with the body's external environment and provides nourishment especially via food, water and air. The Srotas can be treated by needling of the appropriate *marmas/siras* listed in Appendix 1.

Nourishment Channels

Prana/ air

1. Prana Vaha Srotas. The channels which carry Pranic energy or life force into the body. These consist not only of the respiratory system channels buts also includes the large intestine where much Pranic absorption is carried out from food and water. The Pranic or energetic channels are directly related to these channels.

Damaged by: Malnutrition, hyperactivity or hyper-exercise, pollution, smoking.

---

87 Dr. David Frawley *Ayurvedic Healing*. (pp.10, 11).
88 Iyengar, BKS. (p.32).
89 Ama means toxins and undigested food particles.

Food

2. Anna Vaha Srotas. These channels carry food (*anna*) and are mainly the digestive system or g.i. tract (*Mahasrota* or the Great Channel).

Damaged by: Wrong food types, excessive and denatured food, *Jathara Agni* imbalance.

Water

3. Ambhu Vaha Srotas. These are the channels that carry or regulate water (*Ambhu*) metabolism, principally the water absorption quality of the g.i. tract.

Damaged by: Fear, excessive exposure to heat, *ama*, alcohol, excessive dry food.

The 7 Tissue Channels

These are the channels which directly relate to the 7 tissues (*Dhatus*) classification of Ayurveda.

Plasma

4. Rasa Vaha Srotas. The channels which carry plasma (*Rasa*) and are related to the lymphatic and the circulatory systems.

Damaged by: Excessive *Kapha* -increasing food, excessive eating or worrying.

Blood

5. Rakta Vaha Srotas. The channels which carry blood (*Rakta*) and relating to the circulatory system of blood flow, originating in the liver where blood cells are produced (and spleen where they are destroyed).

Damaged by: Over stimulating or hot food and drinks, excess heat (e.g. Sun) (*Pitta* increasing).

Muscle

6. Mamsa Vaha Srotas. The channels which carry nutrients to the muscles (*Mamsa*) thus relating to the muscular system.

Damaged by: *Kapha* increasing diets consisting of heavy substances, excess sleeping.

Fat

7. Medo Vaha Srotas. The channels that supply fat or adipose tissue (*medas*) to the body, originating in the kidneys and abdomen.

Damaged by: Insufficient exercise, excessive sleeping, *Kapha* type food (oily/fatty) in excess.

Bone

8. Asthi Vaha Srotas. The channels that provide nutrients to the bones (*asthi*) and relating to the skeletal system.

Damaged by: *Vata* type diets, strains on joints by excessive jarring or jerking motions.

Marrow/nerve

9. Majja Vaha Srotas. The channels which supply marrow or nerve tissue (*Majja*) to the body and therefore relating to the nervous system and brain. This may be the cerebral-spinal fluid. Its origins are the bones and kidneys.

Damaged by: Physical (and emotional) traumatic injuries, excess noises.

Reproductive tissue

10. Shukra Vaha Srotas. The channels which supply the reproductive tissue (semen and ovum) and hence it is related to the reproductive system in general. It originates in the male testes and female uterus.

Damaged by: Surgery (especially scars which block the channels) and chemo/radiotherapy, excess sex or suppression of strong sexual desire.

The third group relates to the channels dealing with the waste material of the body, mainly urine, feces and sweat.

Waste product channels

Sweat

11. Sveda Vaha Srotas. These are the channels which carry perspiration or sweat (*sveda*) and also includes the sebaceous system. It originates in the adipose tissue and hair.

Damaged by: Excessive heat and exercise, excess taking of heating foods, excess anger.

Feces

12. *Purisha Vaha Srotas*. These are the channels that carry feces (*Purisha*) and involves the excretory system, mainly the large intestine and the rectum.

Damaged by: Suppression of desire to defecate, taking of food before the previous meal has been digested, low *Agni* or excessive eating.

Urine

13. *Mutra Vaha Srotas*. These are the channels which carry urine (*Mutra*) and relate to the urinary system, mainly the kidneys and bladder, ureters and urethra.

Damaged by: Incorrect usage of reproductive/urinary organs, trauma to these or excessive traveling which affects the kidneys.

The fourth group is peculiar to the female as it involves and includes the female reproductive system and conception, menstruation and breastfeeding.

Female Reproductive channels

14. Artava Vaha Srotas. These are the channels which regulate and carry menstrual flow (*Artava*) and also includes the female secretions used during sex. They involve the female reproductive system and have their origin in the uterus. The acupuncture Conception channel, *Janma Nadi* has a direct relationship to these channels. *Janma Nadi* originates in the reproductive system and crosses the area of reproduction and conception (uterus).

Damaged by: Excess or deficient sex (if the person desires it), malnourishment and emotions such as fear, anger and grief.

Lactation

15. *Stanya Vaha Srotas*. These are the lactation channels which carry breast milk (*Stanya*) and their origin like the previous female channels (*Artava*) is in the uterus. The acupuncture Conception channel , *Janma Nadi* has a direct relationship to these channels as *Janma Nadi* also crosses the breast area where lactation occurs.

Damaged by: Breast milk suppression or excessive breast feeding.

The last or fifth group relates to the function of the mind which controls the body.

The Mind channels

Mental process

16. Mano Vaha Srotas. These are the channels which carry thought, ideas and emotions and relate to the mental system. It also communicates with the nervous system (for nerve impulse communication) and relate to the motor and sensory nerve systems.

Damaged by: Emotional factors, excess emotions, suppression of emotions, hallucinogenic drugs, excessive strong stimuli (e.g. loud sounds).

Srotas treatment examples

Treatment of the srotas can be performed by needling of the appropriate siras as shown in the examples below. Refer to Appendix 1 for complete listing.

Mind srotas
Minister 20 - G 20 (*adhipati marma*). (major *Vata* sedative point).

Heart 7 - H 7 (*Hridaya sira*) (major *Vata* nerve remote point)

Lactation srotas
Conception 17 - C 17 (*hridaya marma*). Heart point (for agalactia).

Muscle srotas
Spleen 3- Sp 3 (*pliha prithvi sira*). The Base and Earth point of the Spleen also called *Mula Pliha sira.*

Food srotas
Tridosha 9- 3D 9 (*Indrabasti marma*). Increases *Agni* (metabolic fire) in small intestine and allows correct absorption.

Prana vaha srotas
Pericardium 8 - P 8 (*Talahridaya marma*). Heart and lung flow *marma/sira* [Fire point].

Governor 24.5 - G24.5 (*Sthapani marma*). 'third eye' Amatya/Shukra 24.5, Brow chakra, also pituitary function.

Srotas and their treatment siras

No.	Srotas	Siras
1	*Prana Vaha Srotas*	Pericardium 8, Governor 24.5
2	*Anna Vaha Srotas*	Tridosha 9, U.Bladder 57
3	*Ambhu Vaha Srotas*	Conception 3, P2, UB40, LI14
4	*Rasa Vaha Srotas*	Tridosha 9
5	*Rakta Vaha Srotas*	C17, LI18, Stomach 8
6	*Mamsa Vaha Srotas*	Spleen 3
7	*Medo Vaha Srotas*	Conception 2
8	*Asthi Vaha Srotas*	Stomach 8
9	*Majja Vaha Srotas*	Governor 20 (G20), G25, G27
10	*Shukra Vaha Srotas*	Conception 2, G.Bladder 29
11	*Sveda Vaha Srotas*	Liver 2, Liver 3
12	*Purisha Vaha Srotas*	C2, G15, G16
13	*Mutra Vaha Srotas*	UB30, UB36, G.Bladder 29
14	*Artava Vaha Srotas* (female)	Spleen 6, UB30, UB36, GB29
15	*Stanya Vaha Srotas* (female)	Conception 17, Spleen 6
16	*Mano Vaha Srotas*	G20 *Adhipati*, H7 *Hridaya sira*

Some siras having a number of different qualities or properties may relate to more than one of the srotas.

Acute and Chronic Srotas Siras

Interestingly, srotas are also found as points or siras on the rear of the body as well as the front of the torso. Certain points or siras along the Urinary bladder channel (*mutrashaya dhamani*) on the rear of the torso (fig.26) not only reflect the organs (organ siras) but these same ones relate to their srotas. These 12 rear points treat chronic symptoms of their related organs and srotas. For instance, Heart and Pranavaha Srotas we can use UB15, Stomach and Annavaha Srotas UB21, Liver and Raktavaha Srotas UB18 etc.

Similar points are also located on the front of the torso but in this case treat acute symptoms of their related organs and srotas. Please refer to the Appendix for a complete listing.

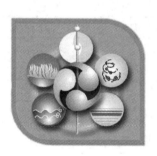

The 107 major marmas

Vital Points (Marmas)

The knowledge of the Ayurvedic 107 major lethal points has been traditionally used in surgery and these were targeted by warriors (*Kshatriyas*) or Indian martial artists. Likewise they were also used by Ayurvedic Acupuncturists (Indian and Sri Lankan etc.) to effect healing not only on humans but also on animals as well, such as the elephant. In Ayurvedic acupuncture we attempt to needle the corresponding sira(s) of the marma with which it has an intricate connection.

It is interesting to note that it was not until recent times, in the last several decades or so that the knowledge of the lethal strike points or marmas had become public knowledge, reluctance to describe them and their locations was usual but after a number of publications, this knowledge is now in the public domain. An attempt to discover if these points were the same in India and the Orient was carried out as explained by Reid and Croucher.

> " Experts, who have compared the locations of the vital spots revealed in ancient Indian texts with the locations known to practitioners of the modern Chinese and Japanese [martial] arts, have found a high degree of correlation." [90]

90 Reid H., Croucher M. *The Way of the Warrior*. Century Publishing, London. 1985. (p.57).

Physical components

According to Ayurveda, a *marma* is the site of *Prana* on the surface of the body also a site of concentration of a number of physical tissues, although it is not always necessary for all these to be present to constitute a *marma*.

These tissues include:

1	bone (*Asthi*)
2	muscle (*Mamsa*)
3	ligament (*Snayu*)
4	nerve (*Majja*)
5	blood vessels (*Shira*)
6	joints (*Sandhi*)

Marmas are also the sites of *Sattva*, *Rajas* and *Tamas* or three psychological energies as well as of *Vata*, *Pitta* and *Kapha*, the three humoral energies (Bishagratna, p.189).

Sushruta was the ancient surgeon who utilized very advanced surgical techniques since Indian surgery was considered then the most advanced in the world. In the *Sushruta Samhita*, a text which appears to have been written at about the time of the Buddha (500 BC) and credited to Sushruta himself, there are a number of chapters dealing with surgery, surgical instruments and the 107 vital lethal points or *marmas*.

> *"Firm unions of Mamsa (muscles) Shira (veins) Sanyo (ligaments),*
> *bones or bone joints are called marmas (or vital parts of the body)*
> *which naturally and specifically form the seats of life (**Prana**), and hence*
> *a hurt to any one of the Marmas invariably produces such symptoms*
> *as arise from the hurt of a certain Marma."* [91]

In Chapter 6, Sushruta commences thus:

> *"Now we shall discourse on the Shariram* which specifically treats*
> *the Marmas or vital parts of the body (places where veins, arteries, ligaments,*
> *joints and muscles unite and an injury to which proves generally fatal).*

> *There are one hundred and seven marmas (in the human organism)*
> *which may be divided into five classes such as Mamsa Marmas [muscle],*
> *Shira Marmas [veins], Sanyo Marmas [ligaments], Asthi Marmas [bone]*
> *and the Sandhi Marmas [joints]."* [92]

---

91 Bishagratna. (p.176).
92 Bishagratna. (p.173).

* [**Note**: *Shariram* means 'body' and consequently refers to the anatomy of the body- in this case the anatomy of the *marmas*].

Marmas are divided into five classes as the location of these *marmas* may lie over a joint, muscle or ligaments etc, or else they lie over a combination of some or all of these. It is because a *marma* may lie over a principal vein or muscle etc. that it may be classified under these types.

So the 107 marmas are not only the lethal points but also those which appear to lie over "*vulnerable or vital parts*" [93] of the body.

> "*Marmas apparently have been known since Vedic times.
> Warriors targeted marmas on their enemies and surgeons employed
> the knowledge of marmas in their treatment of such injuries.*" [94]

Professor Dr. Kulkarni further explains :

> "*Sushruta has advised curved needles for stitches in Marma areas.
> This implies that Sushruta himself has not denied surgery in Marma area.
> Surgery in these areas has to be done when required. We know of many
> successful heart operations although heart is a Marma area.*" [95]

> "*The main difference in surgery or injury and in
> acupuncture is the extent and severity of the injury.*"

and

> "*We know by experience that nothing wrong is going to happen if a needle is
> pricked over the sternum, which is an area of the heart Marma.*" [69]

The 107 lethal *marmas* are for the most part also some of the acupuncture *marmas* today utilized in Ayurvedic acupuncture. Some of the marmas used in acupuncture, which are not classified by Sushruta, are indeed not very lethal if injured by an arrow or such other weapon.

Lethal in this context does not mean 'resulting in death' but rather *causing major harm, which may indeed result in death*. These less lethal marmas are called siras by Sushruta. In this text, siras can also be called marmas interchangeably, unless we are specifically referring to the 107 marmas.

However, all *marmas* or *siras* will cause harm if the appropriate type of injury is applied to them. For instance, a poison injected into a *marma* or sira located in the upper arm may cause irreparable damage to the organ with which the

93 Ibid. (p.173).
94 Svoboda, R. *Ayurveda, Life, Health and Longevity.* (p.65).
95 Kulkarni, P.H. (p.7).

marma directly relates e.g. the large intestine, so that cancer may appear in the colon a number of years after the poison was injected at the *marma*.

> *"The body of a person, hurt in any of the vaikalyakara Marmas, may remain operative only under a skilful medical treatment; but a deformity of the affected organ is inevitable."* [96]

Sushruta's 107 *marmas* exemplified the use of these in surgery and direct harm from *major* trauma. Marmas always contain one or more *siras*, which are related to marmas but are the sensitive spots that can be punctured in siravedhana or Ayurvedic acupuncture. According to Sushruta there are at least 700 of these siras over the entire human body.

These are directly in accordance with what today we call the acupuncture points and which are classified by the W.H.O. under the international numbering system which is today also used in Ayurvedic acupuncture as a form of convention.

Classes
There are five classes of major lethal *marmas*:

1) eleven major *marmas* relate to Muscle (*Mamsa*)

2) forty-one *marmas* relate to Veins (*Sira*)

3) twenty-seven *marmas* relate to Ligaments (*Snayu*)

4) eight major *marmas* relate to Bone (*Asthi*)

5) twenty *marmas* relate to Joints (*Sandhi*).

General Location
These *marmas* are located as follows:

a) Twenty-two (22) in the legs

b) Twenty-two (22) in the arms

c) Twelve (12) front of torso

d) Fourteen (14) rear of torso

e) Thirty-seven (37) in the head and neck area.

Names of Marmas
The names of these *marmas* are often repeated so that a *marma* may be called *Kurccha* on the arm and another *marma* may be likewise called *Kurccha* but is

---

96 Bishagratna. (p.190).

located on the leg. This produces a complication and so often the term *Pada* (foot) is prefixed to *Kurccha* to denote it is located in the leg, not the arm. For example- *Pada Kurccha Marma*.

In Ayurvedic acupuncture this terminology may often cause complications and hence some of these *marmas* are likewise referred to by other names so as not to confuse the issue. A *marma* may be referred to by different terms and still denoting the same *marma*. Where possible, the Sushruta traditional names should be used.

It is generally believed that the overall concept of discouraging the use of acupuncture on the 107 *marmas* was developed in India to attempt to hide the concepts and system of Ayurvedic acupuncture from the populace, as a form of protection for those who practiced it as well as for the system in general, especially so during periods of domination of India by foreign powers. Also, it was to ensure that unqualified people did not needle these susceptible points which should only be treated by the experts.

Dangerous Marmas
There are a number of major lethal *marmas* that are not normally needled in Ayurvedic acupuncture as they are considered extremely dangerous and thus prohibited. These include the *marmas* on the nipple and navel.

Lethal Qualitative Classifications
Marmas are also divided into five classes according to their lethal effects. These five directly relate to the Five Elements.

The following classifications will be used in the text to follow.

PROGNOSIS
Marmas when injured may cause:

Sadya marmas

① **fatality within twenty-four hours.** This is due to the *marmas'* direct connection with the **Fire** Element as fire is easily enfeebled.

Kalantara marmas

② **fatality within a fortnight or month.** This is due to the *marmas'* direct connection to the **Fire** and **Water** Elements as these two elements (especially Water) allow the trauma to linger on before finally succumbing to death.

Vishalyaghna marmas

③ **fatality when the offending sharp object** (shalya) **is removed.** This is due to the *marmas'* direct connection to the Wind Element as **Wind** or Air (and *Prana*) tends to escape if the object is removed, causing death.

Vaikalyakara marmas

④ **maiming or deforming effect to the limb or connecting organ.** This is due to the *marmas'* connection to the **Water** Element that tends to deform the organism.

Rujakar marmas

⑤ **extremely painful sensations when injured.** This is due to the *marmas'* connection to the **Fire** and **Wind** Elements since these two tend to generate pain.

Muscle Marmas (Mamsa Marmas)

Tala Hridaya Marma (upper)
Location: palm
Sira Number: P8
Prognosis: ② fatal within a fortnight or month.
Effect: extreme pain that may result in death. Cardiac pain.
Therapy: stimulates the lungs (*Vata*).

Tala Hridaya Marma (lower)
Location: sole of foot
Sira Number: K1
Prognosis: ② fatal within a fortnight or month.
Effect: extreme pain that may result in death. Cardiac pain.
Therapy: stimulates the kidneys (*Vata*).

Indra Basti Marma (upper)
Location: middle of forearm
Sira Number: P4, L6, 3D9
Prognosis: ② fatal within a fortnight or month.
Effect: excessive hemorrhage that may result in death.
Therapy: stimulates *Agni*, the digestive intestinal 'Fire'.

Indra Basti Marma (lower)
Location: middle of calf
Sira Number: UB57
Prognosis: ② fatal within a fortnight or month.
Effect: excessive hemorrhage that may result in death.
Therapy: stimulates *Agni*, the digestive intestinal 'Fire'.

Guda Marma
Location: located in perineal area, connected with the large intestine, controlling stool and flatulence.
Sira Number: Minister1, Conception 1 (G1,C1)
Prognosis: ① fatal within twenty-four hours.
Effect: if injured may result in death. This is the same area as the Earth Chakra.
Therapy: stimulates uro-genito functions. This is also the local *Apana Vayu sira* on the torso.

Stanya Rohita
Location: located 2 *angulis* above the nipples.
Sira Number: Sp20
Prognosis: ② fatal after a fortnight or month.
Effect: fills thoracic cavity with blood with much coughing and difficulty in breathing that may result in death.
Therapy: sedates the arms.

Vein Marmas (Shira Marmas)

Nila Dhamani Marma
Location: located on throat near beginning of sternum.
Sira Number: St9, LI18
Prognosis: ④ maiming or deforming.
Effect: causes dumbness, loss of taste and aphonia. Injury may result in death.
Therapy: balances the sense of timing and treats aphonia and loss of taste.

Matrika Marma- Kantha Siras
Location: located either side of neck.
Sira Number: GB21, 3D16, LI17, G15, C23
Prognosis: ① fatal within twenty-four hours.
Effect: may result in death.
Therapy: may assist in the flow of blood in the head.

Shringataka Marma
Location: on nose, top lip, chin area.
Sira Number: (1) GB4, St8, UB4; (2) GB15, UB5, G22, M23
Prognosis: ① fatal within twenty-four hours.
Effect: generally soothes the eyes, ears, nose and tongue and which if injured may result in death.
Therapy: stimulates the nervous system and soothes the eyes, ears, nose and tongue.

Apanga Marma
Location: corner of eyes.
Sira Number: GB1, 3D23
Prognosis: ④ maiming or deforming.
Effect: blindness or defective vision.
Therapy: reduces nervous stress and may treat defective vision.

Sthapani Marma
Location: center of head, between eyebrows.
Sira Number: Extra point G24.5
Prognosis: ③ fatal if a sharp object is removed from the injured *marma*, the patient remaining alive while the shaft is left in place.
Effect: related to the pituitary gland and a major site of *Prana*. Location of the Brow Chakra.
Therapy: balances the mind and the nervous system including the Pituitary gland.

Phana Marma
Location: attached to interior channels of both nostrils.
Sira Number: LI19, LI20
Prognosis: ④ maiming or deforming.
Effect: loss of smell.
Therapy: runny nose, nasal obstruction, and nosebleeds.

Stana Mula Marma
Location: nipples, also directly below nipples.
Sira Number: Sp17, St18, K22
Prognosis: ② fatal after a fortnight or month.
Effect: fills thorax with *Kapha*, causing coughs and difficult breathing.
Therapy: not needled. Assists in coughs and apnea.

Apalapa Marma
Location: in the axillary area
Sira Number: L1
Prognosis: ② fatal within a fortnight or month.
Effect: transforms blood into pus that may result in death.
Therapy: balances the sympathetic and parasympathetic nervous systems.

Apastambha Marma
Location: center between the nipple and the collarbone.
Sira Number: Sp19
Prognosis: ② fatal after a fortnight or month.
Effect: fills thoracic cavity with *Vayu* and causes coughing and dyspepsia that may result in death.
Therapy: asthma, coughs and dyspepsia

Hridaya Marma
Location: center of thorax, middle of sternum.
Sira Number: C17. (Hridaya as an organ has C14-C15 as siras).
Prognosis: ① fatal within twenty-four hours.
Effect: seat of *Sattva, Rajas* and *Tamas*, breast disease and affects the circulation and breathing.
Therapy: controls the centrifugal Pranic flow (*Vyana Vayu*), breast disease, allows balance in circulation and breathing. Affects *Sadhaka Pitta* that causes fantasies and realities to become indistinguishable when vitiated. May treat the Pericardium organ.

Nabhi Marma
Location: navel.
Sira Number: C8
Prognosis: ① fatal within twenty-four hours.
Effect: injury results in death. Not needled in Ayurvedic acupuncture.
Therapy: not needled but when massaged may stimulate the small intestine and *Pachaka Pitta*. May treat hyperacidity and gastric, duodenal ulcers. *Nabhi* is the junction of all the *Siras* (arteries/veins) and major inlet of *Prana* into the body according to some authorities.

Parshva Sandhi Marma
Location: rear of torso about hip level.
Sira Number: GB26
Prognosis: ② fatal within a fortnight or month.
Effect: fills abdominal cavity with blood that may result in death.
Therapy: assists circulation.

Vrihati Marma
Location: between spine and shoulder blade at the level of the heart.
Sira Number: UB47, UB18
Prognosis: ② fatal within a fortnight or month.
Effect: excessive loss of blood that may result in death.
Therapy: coughing of blood, heart symptoms.

Lohitaksha Marma
Location: center of the armpits and of the groin (crease)
Sira Number: H1, Lv11
Prognosis: ④ maiming or deforming.
Effect: causes excessive bleeding and creates paralysis of the leg or arm.
Therapy: assists circulation and pain in limbs.

Urvi Marma (upper)
Location: situated in the center of the upper arm.
Sira Number: P2
Prognosis: ④ maiming or deforming.
Effect: atrophy of arm due to causative excessive bleeding.
Therapy: stimulates *Ambhu Vaha Srotas*, urine retention and swelling and pain in axillary area.

Urvi Marma (lower)
Location: situated in the center of the thigh.
Sira Number: St32, UB37
Prognosis: ④ maiming or deforming.
Effect: atrophy of leg due to causative excessive bleeding.
Therapy: stimulates *Ambhu Vaha Srotas*, urine retention and swelling and pain in inguinal area.

Ligament Marmas (Snayu Marmas)

Ani Marma (upper)
Location: approximately three *angulis* above the elbow joint.
Sira Number: LI12, 3D11, L4
Prognosis: ④ maiming or deforming.
Effect: causes numbness and paralysis of the leg or arm.
Therapy: controls muscle tone.

Ani Marma (lower)
Location: approximately three *angulis* above the knee joint.
Sira Number: GB31, St33, Lv9, Sp10

Prognosis: ④ maiming or deforming.
Effect: causes numbness and paralysis of the leg or arm.
Therapy: controls muscle tone.

Vitapa Marma
Location: between scrotum and inguinal region on leg.
Sira Number: K11
Prognosis: ④ maiming or deforming.
Effect: produces infertility and impotence.
Therapy: impotence, urine retention, external genital pain, and seminal emission. Affects muscle tone in lower abdomen.

Kakshadhara Marma
Location: located in the joint between arm and chest.
Sira Number: 3D14
Prognosis: ④ maiming or deforming.
Effect: may result in hemiplegia.
Therapy:. Affects muscle tone in upper abdomen and chest.

Kurccha Marma
Location: (a) located in web between thumb and index finger and (b) on the center of the thumb pad, palm side of hand.
Sira Number: LI5, 3D3
Prognosis: ④ maiming or deforming.
Effect: results in incorrect positioning of the hand and also causes shivering. This marma deals with Vata- the Large Intestine and the Lung.
Therapy: treatment of the large intestine, pain.

Pada Kurccha Marma
Location: 2 *angulis* from web of big toe and first toe.
Sira Number: GB42, Lv3
Prognosis: ④ maiming or deforming.
Effect: shaking and incorrect positioning of foot.
Therapy: high blood pressure, jaundice, uterine bleeding.

Kurccha Shira Marma
Location: located (a) on the thumb area of the wrist crease both on the inside and outside surfaces (b) on the little finger area, inside and outside of the wrist.
Sira Number: 3D4, SI5
Prognosis: ④ maiming or deforming.
Effect: spasm, pain and swelling of the wrist.
Therapy: heart and lung symptoms.

Pada Kurccha Shira Marma
Location: located on the inside and outside of the ankle joint.
Sira Number: Sp5, St42
Prognosis: ④ maiming or deforming.
Effect: pain and swelling of the ankle.
Therapy: leg and back ache, epilepsy.

Basti Marma
Location: located front, center of body, in the groin area.
Sira Number: C3-6, UB28
Prognosis: ② fatal within twenty-four hours.
Effect: treatment of this *marma* assists in stimulating *Kapha*.
Therapy: genito-urinary disorders.

Kshipra Marma
Location: located at the commencement of the web formed between the thumb and index finger.
Sira Number: LI4
Prognosis: ② fatal within a fortnight or month.
Effect: convulsions that may result in death.
Therapy: eye pain, toothache, redness and pain in fingers.

Pada Kshipra Marma
Location: located at the commencement of the web formed between the big toe and first toe (a) on top of foot and (b) sole.
Sira Number: Lv2, Lv3
Prognosis: ② fatal within a fortnight or month.
Effect: convulsions that may result in death.
Therapy: swelling, redness and pain in eye and toes.

Amsa Marma
Location: located center of shoulder, between spine and end of shoulder.
Sira Number: GB21
Prognosis: ④ maiming or deforming.
Effect: incapacity to move arm. Hormonal system *marma* and affecting the throat.
Therapy: stimulates Throat chakra, thyroid and the endocrine system.

Vidhura Marma
Location: directly below the ear.
Sira Number: 3D16, 3D17
Prognosis: ④ maiming or deforming.
Effect: loss of hearing, movement of head.
Therapy: ear disorders, facial paralysis.

Utkshepa Marma
Location: located at temporal area on hairline.
Sira Number: Extra point by side of St8
Prognosis: ③ fatal when weapon is removed.
Effect: removal of injuring object may result in death. Stimulates the large intestine.
Therapy: temporal headaches.

Bone Marmas (Asthi Marmas)

Katika Taruna Marma
Location: located at the joint of the sacrum-illeum articulation.
Sira Number: UB31, UB53
Prognosis: ② fatal within a fortnight or month.
Effect: excessive hemorrhaging leading to pallor of skin which may result in death.
Therapy: treatment of hip joint.

Nitamva Marma
Location: side, above pelvis.
Sira Number: GB29
Prognosis: ② fatal within a fortnight or month.
Effect: atrophy and weakness in extremities that may result in death.
Therapy: low backache, sciatica, paralysis of lower limb, large intestine problems.

Amsaphalaka Marma
Location: located side of vertebral column, start of shoulder blade.
Sira Number: UB11, UB41
Prognosis: ④ maiming or deforming.
Effect: results in atrophy/ loss of sensation of the arm.
Therapy: scapular pain and fourth chakra treatment (chest).

Shankha Marma
Location: located at the junction of the frontal, sphenoid and temporal bones (outside end of eyebrows).

Sira Number: Extra point (between top of ear and outer end of eyebrow) (vicinity of GB4-GB5)
Prognosis: ① fatal within twenty-four hours.
Effect: may result in death.
Therapy: treats hearing, temporal headaches.

Joint Marmas (Sandhi Marmas)

Janu Marma
Location: located at the knee.
Sira Number: GB34, UB40, St35
Prognosis: ④ maiming or deforming.
Effect: results in lameness, especially of the leg and lower back. Assists in stimulating the heart and spleen.
Therapy: treats the lower back and leg pain, including the hip joint.

Kurpara Marma
Location: located in elbow, above the joint.
Sira Number: LI11, SI8, 3D10
Prognosis: ④ maiming or deforming.
Effect: lameness of arm.
Therapy: numbness of arm, elbow pain, cardiac pain, coughs, asthma.

Simanta Marma
Location: located on top of head at suture, between frontal and temporal areas.
Sira Number: Extra points (4) surrounding Adhipati G20
Prognosis: ② fatal within a fortnight or month.
Effect: fear and madness that may result in death. Assists circulation of blood in the head.
Therapy: migraine, lacrimation, and fear.

Adhipati Marma
Location: located on center of top of head.
Sira Number: G20
Prognosis: ① fatal within twenty-four hours.
Effect: results in grave effects to *Prana*, the nervous system that may result in death. This *marma* is extremely useful in the treatment of epilepsy, and psychiatric diseases. It is the major site or gate of *Prana*.
Therapy: treatment of psychiatric diseases and nervous system disorders, Pranic energy balancer, pineal gland and brain disorders.

Gulpha Marma
Location: rear joint of foot and calf.
Sira Number: UB59, GB39
Prognosis: ④ maiming or deforming.
Effect: results in maimness, pain and paralysis of the leg.
Therapy: treatment of leg paralysis and pain (especially in ankle joint).

Manibandha Marma
Location: located at the center of joint of the hand and arm, at the wrist.
Sira Number: SI5, 3D5
Prognosis: ② fatal within a fortnight or month.
Effect: results in motor dysfunction of hand.
Therapy: treats diseases of the wrist, carpal tunnel syndrome, cardiac pain, and mental disorders.

Kukundara Marma
Location: located either side of sacral spine at the sacral sciatic notch.
Sira Number: GB29
Prognosis: ④ maiming or deforming.
Effect: paralysis, loss of sensation of the lower back and leg.
Therapy: Local, rear *Apana Vayu marma*.

Avarta Marma
Location: located at end and slight above of the eyebrows, at approximately the level of *Sthapani marma*.
Sira Number: GB14
Prognosis: ④ maiming or deforming.
Effect: results in impairment of vision and blindness.
Therapy: Eye disease, sinusitis (frontal) and temporal headaches.

Krikatika Marma
Location: located at the join of the start of the cervical vertebrae and edge of cranium just above the rear hairline.
Sira Number: G15, G16
Prognosis: ④ maiming or deforming.
Effect: results in loss of proper functional movement of head and may result in loss of consciousness.
Therapy: neck and shoulder pain.

C= Conception nadi (*Artava nadi*) G= Governing or Minister nadi (*Shukra nadi*).

Locating Marmas

It is sometimes easy to locate a *marma*, as it is either sensitive to pressure or else forms a slightly hollow area on the body. Most *marmas* often exhibit slight or severe pain when pressured by a finger or thumb and thus their location becomes obvious. When there is a disorder in the body, the marmas (siras) which directly relate to this area or organ will reflect sensitivity in synergy with the remote disorder.

Marmas (or siras) can also be located by a measurement. This is a 'finger measurement' or *anguli*. The width of the thumb of the patient (and not of the practitioner) is usually taken as one *anguli*. A *marma* may be located thus, e.g. –

> "2 angulis proximal from web of big toe and first toe. " [97]

for the Pada Kurccha Marma.

The measurement of *anguli* is relative to the patient and not the therapist.

> "Like the Chinese acupuncture points, Marma points are measured by the finger units (Anguli) relative to each individual. Their size is measured by finger inches and their location determined by them." [98]

Today, siras (marmas) can be detected by using a resistance meter (Ohm meter). The area of the sira is usually lower in resistance than the surrounding area where it is located.

---

97 Bishagratna. (p.173).
98 Dr. Subhash Ranade. *Natural Healing Through Ayurveda.* Passage Press. Utah USA (1993) (p. 161).

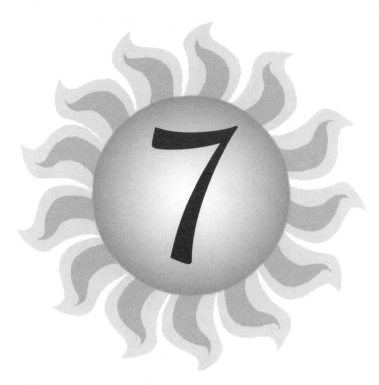

The major acupuncture siras

"All Dhamanis have four types of Siras embedded in their channel.

   10 Vatvaha

   10 Pittavaha

   10 Kaphvaha

   10 Raktavaha

Raktavaha and Pittavaha have their origin in the same channel.

Siras are the points to eradicate disease by puncturing, Agnikarm etc." [99]

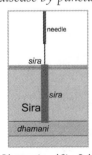

***Fig 13**. Dhamani and Sira Relationship*

99 Drs. R.L.Shah, B.K.Joshi, G.Joshi. *Vedic Health Care System.* (p.31).

Siras are of four types:

- Vatavaha
- Pittavaha
- Kaphavaha
- Raktavaha

Pittavaha and Raktavaha siras have same channel origin (according to Sushruta).

Sushruta explains that there are 700 siras :

- 175 Vatavaha siras (100 extremities/75 torso/head)
- 175 Pittavaha siras (100 extremities/75 torso/head)
- 175 Kaphavaha siras (100 extremities/75 torso/head)
- 175 Raktavaha siras (100 extremities/75 torso/head)

Total 700 siras

There are two channels per one organ, that is each organ has two channels, one on the left hand side of the body and one on the right side of the body. For instance, the Lung channel has one branch down the left arm and one down the right arm, so the number of siras or points must be multiplied by 2.

Vata
Upper extremity:

- Lung channel   (11)
- LI channel   (14)

Total **25** siras x 2 (branches) = 50

Pitta
Upper extremity:

- Heart channel   (9)
- Small intestine channel   (16)

Total **25** siras x 2 (branches) = 50

Kapha
Upper extremity:

- Pericardium channel   (9)
- Tridosha channel (16)

Total **25** siras x 2 (branches) = 50

Vata

Lower extremity:

- Kidney channel   (11)
- Urinary bladder   channel (14)

Total **25** siras x 2 (branches) = 50

Pitta

Lower extremity:

- Liver channel   (12)
- Gall bladder channel   (13)

Total **25** siras x 2 (branches) = 50

Kapha

Lower extremity:

- Spleen channel   (11)
- Stomach channel (14)

Total **25** siras x 2 (branches) = 50

Raktavaha

Extremities:

Total **100** siras = 100

Torso:

- Vatavaha siras   (75)
- Pittavaha siras   (75)
- Kaphavaha siras   (75)
- Raktavaha siras   (75)

Total **300** siras = 300

Total 700 siras

The 700 Siras

"In fact, 24 channels (meridians) are... Sushrut's 24 Dhamanis while [acu]points on channels are 700 Siras of Sushrut. Sushrut has very authentically mentioned that Siras are embedded in Dhamanis other than [the] extra canals [nadis]." [100]

100 Drs. R.L.Shah, B.K.Joshi, G.Joshi. *Vedic Health Care System.* (p.viii).

Sushruta delineated four types of humors- Vata, Pitta, Kapha and Rakta, although Rakta had the same points (siras) as Pitta.

When we check the siras according to the 12 organ channels (*dhamanis*) and the two extra channels (*nadis*)- Artava and Shukra nadis (=14 channels) we also find a number equal to 700 siras, including 30 siras which are classified as *extra points* and sit *outside* of the 14 channels. For instance the 4 siras of Simanta, the sira related to Utkshepa, and others.

Channel	LH	RH	Total
Arm:			
Vata dhamanis			
Lung	(11)	(11)	
LI	(20)	(20)	62
Pitta dhamanis			
S.I.	(19)	(19)	
Heart	(9)	(9)	56
Kapha dhamanis			
Per	(9)	(9)	
3D	(23)	(23)	64
Leg:			
Vata dhamanis			
Kidney	(27)	(27)	
Urinary Bladder	(67)	(67)	188
Pitta dhamanis			
Liver	(14)	(14)	
GB	(44)	(44)	116
Kapha dhamanis			
Stomach	(45)	(45)	
Spleen	(21)	(21)	132

Channel	LH	RH	Total
Nadis			
Shukra nadi (inc. G24.5)	(28)		
Conception (Artava nadi)	(24)		52
Extra siras	(30)		30
		TOTAL	700 siras

Classifications of Siras

In marmapuncture, siras are classified according to their connections' intricacies. There are four types of classifications; hence a sira which connects directly with a marma and its related chakra is classified as a Primary sira because of its complex connections.

Primary

Chakras - Marmas - Siras

Examples: **Chakra   Marma Sira**

- Brow Chakra, *Sthapani* marma, G24.5 Shukra nadi 24.5
- Crown Chakra, *Adhipati* marma, G20 Shukra nadi 20

Secondary

Marmas - Siras

Examples: **Marma Sira**

- *Kshipra* marma   Large Intestine 4
- *Indrabasti* marma Urinary Bladder 57
- *Janu* marma   Urinary Bladder 40

Tertiary
Siras

Special function points, 5 Element points, Bridge points, Base points, Cleft points.

Examples:

5 Element points

- Heart 7 Earth
- Heart 8 Fire
- Heart 9 Ether

Supplementary
Siras

Siras along the channels, having their own individual, unique therapeutic values.

Example:

- Lung 2 asthma and cough, chest pain.

Consequently, siras are present at:

(1) Chakra/marma junctions

(2) Marmas

(3) Singularly at the acupoint also called a sira.

In South India, *siras* are also called *adankals* while in Sri Lanka they are called *nilas*, basically acupoints. Acupoints are not just locations for acupuncture but also for acupressure or any other therapy which may be applicable on the siras (e.g. agnikarma).

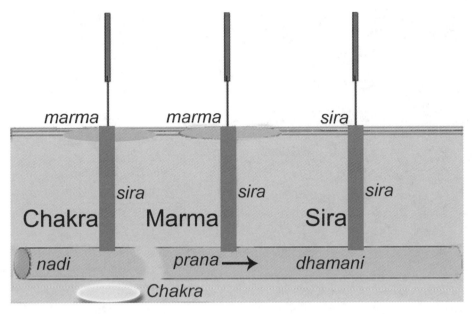

Fig 14. *Chakras, Marmas and Siras*

The 5 element points of ayurvedic acupuncture

Ayurvedic acupuncture/Suchi Karma (*Siravedhana*) explains that each of the twelve organ channels has a number of points which are directly related to the Five Elements (*Pancha Mahabhutas*). These are referred to as the Five Flow Points or Five Sru Points (*Pancha Sru Siras*) (or *Pancha Mahabhutas Siras*) and there are five points on each of the channels which reflect the five elements. These five flow points reflect the effect of Prana based on the organs and elements and consequently when an element (such as Wind/Air) is impaired somewhere in the body, the related flow point becomes tender to the touch, which demonstrates an imbalance in the element and possibly the related organ. The flow here refers to the flow of effect (therapeutic or of malady) and not the flow direction of Prana through the channel.

They are used in treating imbalances caused by the Five Elements but as will be seen, they are an integral part of Ayurvedic knowledge, especially of Suchi Karma (needling therapy) and are extremely important in major therapy. Some of these points are likewise classified under the lethal scheme of Ayurveda, as for instance, *Kurccha Marma* and *Kurccha sira* is Liver 3 or the Stream/Earth point of the Liver Channel.

The elements are reflected along points on the channel according to the **Wheel of Support** of the Five Elements:

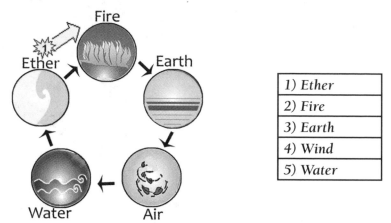

1) *Ether*
2) *Fire*
3) *Earth*
4) *Wind*
5) *Water*

Fig 15. *The Five Elements' Wheel of Support*

However, the first element reflected on the first point along the channel from tip of finger or toe back towards elbow or knee depends on the type of channel it is. All solid organ channels always have Ether as their first element point. All hollow organ channels have Wind as their first element point. Nevertheless, each channel follows the Wheel of Support.

Solid Organ Channels   Hollow Organ Channels

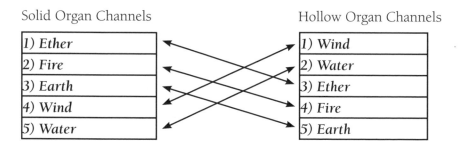

Examples: Solid Organs: Heart, Liver.

Hollow Organs: Bladder, Large Intestine.

The Five Element Points always *start at the fingertips or the ends of the toes and terminate near the elbows or knees in each of the twelve major channels.*

Generically, these five points in all of the twelve channels are called:

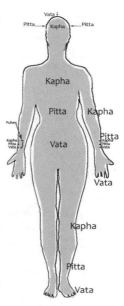

- Well (Kupa)
- Spring (Sara)
- Stream (Sarit)
- River (Dhuni)
- Sea (Samudra)

The Well points have a more subtle effect, akin to Vata or treat more subtle problems (e.g. insomnia) are located near the fingertips or toes. The Spring points akin to Pitta treat slightly more physical problems like inflammation while the Sea points akin to Kapha have a more physical effect, or treat more physical problems (e.g. congestion of the lung, arthritis) and are located near the elbows or knees (according to the channel in question).

Fig.16. VPK locations

These generic terms reflect the flow of *Prana* (the energy of flow) and of Water (the element of flow). When vapor in clouds condenses, it falls to the ground causing a well to be developed. As more water falls, the *well* becomes a *spring*, then a *stream*, a *river* which then flows to the sea, the most physical of all the five.

These generic terms for the Five Sru points reflect only the *effects of subtle to physical (well to sea) which the points treat* and is <u>not necessarily the direction of flow of Prana through the particular channel</u>, this is an important fact which must be realized.

PLEASE NOTE: All Five Element points are located somewhere between the elbows or knees and fingers or toes, respectively and are not to be found in the torso or head areas. These are called *distal* or *remote* points because they exist in the extremities and not the head or torso.

Direction of Pranic flow through the dhamanis differs between channels which results in some channels having the Pranic flow through the channel from the Sea to the Well points (e.g. heart channel) and others from the Well points to the Sea points (Large Intestine channel). The direction of Pranic flow along each channel has been referred to previously and is according to the Pranic Mandala.

The Five Elements

As previously described in the text, the first recorded use of the Five Elements (Pancha Mahabhutas)[Five Great Elements] is in the Vedas. Through Buddhism, these five extended throughout the Orient, first into China and later into Japan.

In Buddhism, the Ether element is called Void, Space or Sky. In Japan the five elements: *godai*, lit. 'five great' are exactly like the Vedic five elements, Earth, Water, Fire, Air and Sky/Void. In China, two names were changed, Wood for Ether and Metal for Air/Wind. These 60 points, the Five Element Points form the nexus or core of acupuncture.

> *"Tsou Yen (c.305-240 BC) tried to amalgamate ideas of Chinese origin with new Western notions which he probably received from Indian travelers. In so doing, he introduced an important innovation[to China and the East], that of the five elements (wu-hing) and their gyration, and of the reciprocal destruction and genesis of these five natural agents."* [101]

It is evident that the Vedic Five Elements and their cycles of creation (*genesis*), destruction, support and control (*gyration*) were adopted ('borrowed') by the Chinese through Buddhism.

> *"From this period onwards, China borrowed from India and Iran. Thus, Tsou Yen introduced to the Far East the idea of the five elements."* [102]

VATA (WIND)

Sru Points of the Lung Channel

The Lung channel has five points along its trajectory which reflect the Five Elements and consequently are called the Five Element Points (*Pancha Mahabhutas Siras*) or (*Pancha Sru Siras*).

1) The first point at the base of the *thumb* is the *Well* point. This point reflects the element of **Ether**, as the Lung is a solid organ. This point is named Lung 11 which means that it is the last point along the *dhamani* of the Lung. The first point of the Lung channel (Lung 1) commences at the chest.

2) The second point is the **Fire** point or *Spring* point, it corresponds with Lung 10 also called *kurccha sira* (on the palm side of hand).

3) The third point is the **Earth** point or *Stream* point, it corresponds to Lung 9.

4) The fourth point is the **Wind** point or *River* point, corresponding to Lung 8.

5) The fifth point is the **Water** point or *Sea* point, corresponding to Lung 5.

101 Prof. P. Huard and Dr. M. Wong. *Chinese Medicine*. World University Press, London. UK. (pp. 88, 89).
102 *Ibid.* (p.12).

Sru Points of the Large Intestine Channel

Like the Lung channel, the Large Intestine channel has five Sru points which reflect the Five Elements. Due to this organ being a hollow organ, the L.I. channel's first point starts with Wind/Air (instead of Ether) and then follows the Wheel of Support (*Alamba Chakra*).

No.	Type	Element	Point No.	Location
1	*Well* Point	**Wind**	Large Intestine 1	Corner of index finger nail
2	*Spring* Point	**Water**	Large Intestine 2.	
3	*Stream* Point	**Ether**	Large Intestine 3	
4	*River* Point.	**Fire**	Large Intestine 5	
5	*Sea* Point.	**Earth**	Large Intestine 11	Outside area of elbow

Humoral significance

These two channels' inter-relationship and connection with the Five Elements and their *Sru* points (as above) allows the development and support of the three humors along the arm.

Vata

So that by taking the first *Well* points of both of these related channels we have:

Lung channel- **Ether**

LI channel- **Wind**

which when combined produce the humoral energy of *Vata* (Ether + Wind). These two points reflect Vata and if needled together will balance this humor.

Pitta

The second set of points (*Spring*) reflects:

Lung channel- **Fire**

L. Intestine channel- **Water**

which combined produce the humoral energy of *Pitta* (Fire + Water). These two points reflect Pitta and if needled together will balance this humor.

Kapha

The fifth set of points (*Sea*) reflects:

Lung channel- **Water**

L. Intestine channel- **Earth**

which combined together produce the humoral energy of *Kapha* (Water + Earth). These two points reflect Kapha and if needled together will balance this humor.

Please note that the third and fourth set of points (Stream and River) do not form individual humors but do have an effect on the humors such as River-Wind/Fire (e.g. hot wind) affecting both Pitta and Vata, while the Stream points - Earth / Ether (e.g. hot sand) affect both Kapha and Pitta.

The above scheme of each pair of element points affecting a humor *applies to all the other paired channels* such as heart/s.intestine, stomach/spleen etc.

KAPHA (EARTH)

Sru Points of the Stomach Channel

The Stomach channel has five points along its trajectory which reflect the Five Elements. These are called the Five Element Points (*Pancha Sru Siras*).

1) The first point at the base of the <u>second toe</u> is the *Well* point. This point reflects the element of **Wind**, as the Stomach is a hollow organ. This point is named Stomach 45 which means that it is the last point along the *dhamani* of the stomach. The first point of the Stomach channel (Stomach 1) commences at the middle, below the bottom eyelid.

2) The second point is the **Water** point or *Spring* point, it corresponds to Stomach 44 .

3) The third point is the **Ether** point or *Stream* point, it corresponds to Stomach 43.

4) The fourth point is the **Fire** point or **River** point, corresponding to Stomach 41.

5) The fifth point is the **Earth** point or *Sea* point, corresponding to Stomach 36.

Sru Points of the Spleen Channel

Like the Stomach channel, the Spleen channel reflects Kapha and the element of Earth and has also five Sru points which reflect the Five Elements. Due to this organ being a solid organ, the Spleen channel's first point starts with Ether (instead of Wind) and then follow the Wheel of Support (Alamba Chakra).

No.	Type	Element	Point	Location
1	*Well Point*	**Ether**	Spleen 1	Corner of large toe nail
2	*Spring Point*	**Fire**	Spleen 2	
3	*Stream Point*	**Earth**	Spleen 3	
4	*River Point*	**Wind**	Spleen 5	
5	*Sea Point*	**Water**	Spleen 9	Inside area of knee

Humoral significance

The Five Sru points of the Stomach and Spleen channels conjointly form the Tridoshas VPK along the leg between these two related channels, which can be needled to treat imbalances in these three humoral energies. Treatment of Kapha on these channels' Sru points is most appropriate (e.g. both Sea points).

PITTA (FIRE)

Sru Points of the Heart Channel

The Heart channel has five points along its trajectory which reflect the Five Elements and called the Five Element Points (Pancha Sru *Siras*).

1) The first point at the inner corner of the <u>little finger</u> is the *Well* point.

This point reflects the element of **Ether**, as the Heart is a solid organ. This point is named Heart 9 which means that it is the last point along the Heart channel. The first point of the Heart channel (Heart 1) commences at the chest.

2) The second point is the **Fire** point or *Spring* point, it corresponds with Heart 8.

3) The third point is the **Earth** point or *Stream* point, it corresponds to Heart 7.

4) The fourth point is the **Wind** point or *River* point, corresponding to Heart 4.

5) The fifth point is the **Water** point or *Sea* point, corresponding to Heart 3.

Sru Points of the Small Intestine Channel

The Small Intestine channel has five Sru points which reflect the Five Elements. Due to this organ being a hollow organ, the S.I. channel's first point starts with Wind (instead of Ether) and then follow the Wheel of Support (Alamba Chakra).

No.	Type	Element	Point	Location
1	Well Point	Wind	Small Intestine 1	Corner of index finger nail
2	Spring Point	Water	Small Intestine 2	
3	Stream Point	Ether	Small Intestine 3	
4	River Point	Fire	Small Intestine 5	
5	Sea Point	Earth	Small Intestine 8	Outside area of elbow

Humoral significance

The Five Sru points of the Heart and Small Intestine channels conjointly form the Tridoshas (VPK) along the arm between these two related channels, which can be needled to treat imbalances in these humoral energies. Treatment of Pitta on these channels' Sru points is most appropriate (e.g. both Spring points).

VATA (WATER -)

Sru Points of the Urinary Bladder Channel

Five Element points (*Pancha Sru Siras*) are reflected along the trajectory of the Urinary Bladder channel.

1) The first point reflects the element of **Wind**, as the Bladder is a hollow organ. This point is Urinary Bladder 67 which means that it is the last point along the channel of the Urinary Bladder. The first point of the U. Bladder channel (UB 1) commences at the inside corner of the eye (lid).

2) The second point is the **Water** point or *Spring* point, it corresponds to UB 66.

3) The third point is the **Ether** point or *Stream* point, it corresponds to UB 65.

4) The fourth point is the **Fire** point or *River* point, corresponding to UB 60.

5) The fifth point is the **Earth** point or *Sea* point, corresponding to UB 40.

Sru Points of the Kidney Channel

Five Sru points reflect the Five Elements along the Kidney channel. Due to this organ being a solid organ, the Kidney channel's first point starts with Ether (instead of Wind) and then follow the Wheel of Support (Alamba Chakra).

No.	Type	Element	Point	Location
1	*Well* Point	**Ether**	Kidney 1	Middle of sole
2	*Spring* Point	**Fire**	Kidney 2	Inside edge of foot
3	*Stream* Point	**Earth**	Kidney 3	Ankle
4	*River* Point	**Wind**	Kidney 7	
5	*Sea* Point	**Water**	Kidney 10	Knee

Humoral significance

The Five Sru points of the Kidney and Urinary Bladder channels conjointly form the Tridoshas (VPK) along the leg between these two related channels, which can be needled to treat imbalances in these humoral energies. Treatment of Vata on these channels' Sru points is most appropriate (e.g. both Well points).

KAPHA (WATER +)

Sru Points of the Pericardium Channel

The Pericardium channel has five points along its trajectory which reflect the Five Elements. These are called the Five Element Points (*Pancha Sru Siras*).

1) The first point at the base of the <u>middle finger</u> is the *Well* point. This point reflects the element of **Ether**, as the Pericardium is a solid organ. This point is named Pericardium 9 which means that it is the last point along the Pericardium channel. The first point of the Pericardium channel (P 1) commences at the chest.

2) The second point is the **Fire** point or *Spring* point, it corresponds with Pericardium 8.

3) The third point is the **Earth** point or *Stream* point, it corresponds to Pericardium 7.

4) The fourth point is the **Wind** point or *River* point, corresponding to Pericardium 5.

5) The fifth point is the **Water** point or *Sea* point, corresponding to Pericardium 3.

The Pericardium channel deals with the balance or flow of the Trigunas or mental energies or 'humors', just like the Tridosha deals with the Tri-doshas or three physical energies. The five Tanmatras (or subtle elements in the mind) are affected by these five Pericardium channel's Sru points. By needling the appropriate element point in this channel, a balance can be obtained in that subtle element or quality in the mind. E.g. by needling the Spring point (**Fire**), correct digestion or formation of ideas can be obtained as fire assists in the formation of things. Likewise, needling of the **Water** point (Sea point), correct flow of ideas can be attained (as Water deals with flow). The Earth (Stream) point attains correct groundness of ideas or thoughts, when this point is needled.

The qualities of the physical elements are mirrored in the psychological elements and their appropriate needling in the Pericardium channel balances these subtle qualities.

Five Elements in the Mind
Ether- provides separation of ideas, gives space between them so that they don't form a clump.

Wind/Air- provides inward direction of ideas into the mind.

Fire- provides digestion and metabolization of ideas into new thoughts or ideas.

Water- provides flow for the ideas within the mind.

Earth- provides an anchor or steadfastness for the ideas so they are not just fleeting thoughts.

Sru Points of the Tridosha Channel
Like the Pericardium channel, the Tridosha channel has five Sru points which reflect the Five Elements. Due to this organ being a hollow organ, the Tridosha channel's first point starts with Wind (instead of Ether) and then follow the Wheel of Support (Alamba Chakra).

No.	Type	Element	Point	Location
1	Well Point	**Wind**	Tridosha 1	Corner of ring-finger nail
2	Spring Point	**Water**	Tridosha 2	
3	Stream Point	**Ether**	Tridosha 3	
4	River Point	**Fire**	Tridosha 6	
5	Sea Point	**Earth**	Tridosha 10	Outside area of elbow

Needling of the five Sru points on the Tridosha channel achieves balance in the physical elements or physical qualities of the body.

Combination of Sru points on the Pericardium and Tridosha channels assists in treating the appropriate humors such as Vata (Well), Pitta (Spring) or Kapha (Sea).

Individual needling assists the *physical* elements (Tridosha channel) and *subtle* elements (Pericardium/Trigunas channel) as well as their related organs (e.g. Fire point- Heart or Small Intestine)

Humoral significance
The Five Sru points of the Pericardium and Tridosha channels conjointly form the Tridoshas along the arm between these two related channels, which can be needled to treat imbalances in these three humoral energies (and three mental energies or Trigunas- via the Pericardium). Treatment of Kapha/flow problems on these channels' Sru points is most appropriate (e.g. both Sea points).

PITTA (ETHER)

Sru Points of the Gall Bladder Channel
The five points along the trajectory of the Gall Bladder channel reflect the Five Elements and are called the Five Element Points (Pancha Sru *Siras*).

1) The first point at the outside corner of the fourth toe is the *Well* point. This point reflects the element of **Wind**, as the Gall Bladder is a hollow organ. This point is named Gall Bladder 44 which means that it is the last point along the Gall Bladder channel. *The first point of the G.B. channel (GB 1) commences at the outside corner of the eye.*

2) The second point is the **Water** point or *Spring* point, it corresponds with Gall Bladder 43

3) The third point is the **Ether** point or *Stream* point, it corresponds to Gall Bladder 41.

4) The fourth point is the **Fire** point or *River* point, corresponding to Gall Bladder 38.

5) The fifth point is the **Earth** point or *Sea* point, corresponding to Gall Bladder 34.

Sru Points of the Liver Channel

The Liver channel has five points which reflect the Five Elements. This organ is a solid organ, so the first Sru point along the Liver channel starts with Ether (instead of Wind) and then follows the Wheel of Support (Alamba Chakra).

No.	Type	Element	Point	Location
1	*Well* Point	**Ether**	Liver 1	Corner of big toe nail
2	*Spring* Point	**Fire**	Liver 2	
3	*Stream* Point	**Earth**	Liver 3	
4	*River* Point	**Wind**	Liver 4	
5	*Sea* Point	**Water**	Liver 8	Inside of leg just above knee

Humoral significance

The Five Sru points conjointly form the Tridoshas along the leg between the humor's two related channels, which can be needled to treat imbalances in these three humoral energies. Treatment of Pitta on these two channels' Sru points is most appropriate (e.g. both Spring points).

Although Pitta can be treated at the Spring points of any two related channels, the most appropriate ones are the Spring points of the Liver and Gall Bladder channels or Heart and Small Intestine channels. These depend on which part of the body is affected, which humor is aggravated and which time of day/night the symptoms greatly manifest.

The Bhuta Agnis

The bhuta agnis are five fires which transform the five elements within the liver. These metabolize the elements from outside the body (macrocosm) into elements that can be properly used inside the body (microcosm) in much the same way the body metabolizes vitamins etc from vegetables into vitamins that the body can use, since a carrot is not a human but can support him or her through its nutrients being metabolized in the body.

The five bhuta agnis have five specific siras which relate to them and by which we can treat these agnis. These are the Five Element points of the liver dhamani recently discussed in this chapter.

Liver 1 relates to the Ether bhuta-agni through its Ether qualities, likewise, Liver 2 relates to the Fire bhuta-agni through its Fire qualities. Liver 3 relates to the Earth bhuta-agni since it relates to the Earth element and so forth.

No.	Type	Element	Point	BhutaAgnis
1	*Well* Point	**Ether**	Liver 1	*Ether*
2	*Spring* Point	**Fire**	Liver 2	*Fire*
3	*Stream* Point	**Earth**	Liver 3	*Earth*
4	*River* Point	**Wind**	Liver 4	*Wind*
5	*Sea* Point	**Water**	Liver 8	*Water*

The bridge points

Bridge Points (Setu Siras)

Each of the twelve channels of Suchi Karma/ marmapuncture has a point along its trajectory called the Bridge point, Setu sira. Setu means a bridge. This point physically allows a bridge or connection to exist between one channel (dhamani) and its related channel, related by their common element (e.g. heart/ small intestine- Fire).

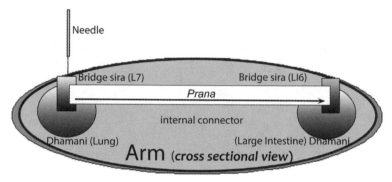

The Minister (Amatya Nadi) [Shukra Nadi] and Conception (Janma Nadi) [Artava Nadi] channels likewise have a related Bridge point each.

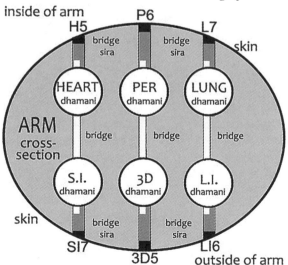

Fig.17. *Bridge points*

The actual bridge itself is an inner channel or duct (not dhamani) which connects with the bridge point on one channel (dhamani) e.g. Lung 7 and with a bridge point on its element-related channel (dhamani) e.g. L. Intestine 6.

Bridge points are usually considered the entrances or gates between the Element-related channels which are linked by a type of energy bridge- thus the term Bridge point. The effect on one channel will recur in its related channel, providing harmony and balance in these two channels.

Treatment of one bridge point of a particular channel, will affect the related channel. For instance, treating the bridge point of the Lung channel, a solid organ channel, will often have a beneficial effect on an imbalance of the Large Intestine, its related hollow organ channel.

Also, by treating the Bridge point, a balance to the particular humor is gained. As with the previous example, the Pranic energy flowing through the Lung / Large Intestine channels will be balanced by treating the bridge points, concurrently balancing Vata in these organs / channels and the areas affected by these.

An additional bridge point exists, located in the Spleen channel which appears to connect with all the other bridge points of the body. It is referred to as the General Bridge point. It acts in much the same manner as the Minister channel (*Shukra Nadi*) 'administers' (*Adhipati*) over the other acupuncture channels (*dhamanis*).

VATA (Wind)

Lung channel Bridge Point
The Lung channel (*Phuphusa dhamani*) has a Bridge point which connects the Lung channel to the Large Intestine channel.

Lung Bridge Point: *Lung 7*   *Setu Phuphusa Sira*

Large Intestine channel Bridge Point
The Large Intestine (*Vrihdantra dhamani*) channel in turn has a Bridge point which connects the Large Intestine channel to the Lung channel.

L.I. Bridge Point: *Large Intestine 6*   *Setu Vrihdantra Sira*

KAPHA (Earth)

Stomach channel Bridge Point
The Stomach channel (*Amashaya dhamani*) has a Bridge point which connects with the Spleen channel.

St. Bridge Point: *Stomach 40*   *Setu Amashaya Sira*

Spleen channel Bridge Point

The Spleen channel (*Pliha dhamani*) inturn has a Bridge point which connects with the Stomach channel.

Sp. Bridge Point: *Spleen 4*   *Setu Pliha Sira*

PITTA (Fire)

Heart channel Bridge Point

The Heart channel (*Hridaya dhamani*) has a Bridge point which connects with the Small Intestine channel.

Heart Bridge Point: *Heart 5*   *Setu Hridaya Sira*

Small Intestine channel Bridge Point

The Small Intestine channel (*Laghvantra dhamani*) in turn has a Bridge point which connects with the Heart channel.

S.I. Bridge Point: *Small Intestine 7*   *Setu Laghvantra Sira*

VATA (Water-)

Urinary Bladder channel Bridge Point

The Urinary Bladder channel (*Mutrashaya dhamani*) has a Bridge point which connects with the Kidney channel.

U.B. Bridge Point: *Urinary Bladder 58*   *Setu Mutrashaya Sira*

Kidney channel Bridge Point

The Kidney channel (Vrikka dhamani) inturn has a Bridge point which connects with the Urinary Bladder channel.

Kidney Bridge Point: *Kidney 4 Setu Vrikka Sira*

KAPHA (Water+)

Pericardium channel Bridge Point

The Pericardium channel (*Talahridaya dhamani*) has a Bridge point which connects with the Tridosha channel.

Per. Bridge Point: *Pericardium 6 Setu Talahridaya Sira*

Tridosha channel Bridge Point

The Tridosha channel (*Tridosha dhamani*) inturn has a Bridge point which connects with the Pericardium channel.

3D Bridge Point: *Tridosha 5*   *Setu Tridosha Sira*

PITTA (Ether)

Gallbladder channel Bridge Point

The Gallbladder channel has a Bridge point which connects with the Liver channel.

GB Bridge Point: *Gallbladder 37Setu Pittashaya Sira*

Liver channel Bridge Point

The Liver channel (*Yakrit dhamani*) inturn has a Bridge point which connects with the Gallbladder channel.

Lv. Bridge Point: *Liver 5*   *Setu Yakrit Sira*

CONCEPTUAL CHANNELS

Conceptual channels relate to the word *concept*- an idea or concept- brain (subtle- governing or minister channel) and conception or birth (physical) -reproductive organs.

Conception channel Bridge Point

The Conception channel (*Artava/Janma Nadi*) has a bridge point which connects this channel with the Minister channel.

Janma Bridge Point: Conception 15   *Setu Artava Sira*

Minister channel Bridge Point

The Minister channel (Amatya/Shukra *Nadi*) likewise has a Bridge point which connects this channel with the Conception channel.

Amatya Bridge Point: Minister 1   *Setu Shukra Sira*

General Bridge Point

The Spleen channel (*Pliha dhamani*) has an additional Bridge point which connects with all the other channels' Bridge points and thereby having an influence or 'ministering' over them.

General Bridge Point: Spleen 21   *Setu Sira*

The base points

The Base Points (Mula Siras)

Each of the twelve organ channels has a base point, *Mula sira*. Mula means a base or root. This is where *Prana* is based along a channel and allowing the energy from the appropriate organ to boost the energy in its related channel.

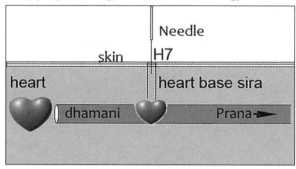

Fig.18. Base point

This may be needed as when a blockage of *Prana* occurs along a channel (as in the case of chronic dis-ease). The Base point will then release energy from the organ into the channel in order to facilitate healing.

The Base point of a channel not only reflects the energy of the related organ but is also a minor doshic representative along the channel. That is to say that in the case of the Lung, the base point of the Lung channel reflects *Vata* in that channel.

Additionally, the Base points reflect the condition of their related organs. For instance an imbalance in the Large Intestine may refer tenderness at Large Intestine 4, at the web between thumb and index finger on the outside of the hand. This knowledge is important as it can be used for diagnosis also, where a device containing an analogue needle meter can be used to measure the resistance at all the Base points, both left side channels of the body and right side channels of the body. The result is fed into a computer for analysis which determines whether an organ is:

- **deficient** (the reading is lower than average)
- **in excess** (the reading is higher than average)
- **unbalanced** (there is a difference in readings between the related left and right channels at their Base points).

Base points generally tend to *treat chronic disorders* best, by re-enforcing the Pranic energy level in the channel and its paired dhamani (e.g. Lung-LI).

* Additionally, the Base points of all the <u>Solid organ channels</u> (only) are also the Stream points of the channels. From this viewpoint, these points also treat imbalances of their respective Elements (e.g.

- *Earth* - solid organ channels) Mula siras

- *Ether* - hollow organ channels). Mula siras

VATA (AM)

The Lung channel Base Point
The Lung channel has a Base point on the inside of the arm. * It also shares the function of being the Stream point of the Lung channel.

Lung Channel Base Point: *Lung 9*   *Mula Phuphusa Sira*

The Large Intestine channel Base Point
The Large Intestine has a Base point on the rear of the arm.

L.I. Channel Base Point: *Large Intestine 4*   *Mula Vrihdantra Sira*

KAPHA (AM)

The Stomach channel Base Point
The Stomach channel has a Base point in the front of the leg.

St. Channel Base Point: *Stomach 42*   *Mula Amashaya Sira*

The Spleen channel Base Point
The Spleen channel has a Base point on the inside of the leg. * It also shares its function as the Stream point of the Spleen channel.

Sp. Channel Base Point: *Spleen 3*   *Mula Pliha Sira*

PITTA (NOON)

The Heart channel Base Point
The Heart channel has a Base point on the inside of the arm. * It shares its function as the Stream point of the Heart channel.

H. Channel Base Point: *Heart 7*   *Mula Hridaya Sira*

The Small Intestine channel Base Point

The Small Intestine channel has a Base point on the outside of the arm.

S.I. Channel Base Point: *Small Intestine 4* *Mula Laghvantra Sira*

VATA (PM)

The Urinary Bladder channel Base Point

The Urinary Bladder has a Base point on the outside edge of the foot.

U.B. Channel Base Point: *Urinary Bladder 64* *Mula Mutrashaya Sira*

The Kidney channel Base Point

The Kidney channel has a Base point on the inside of the leg, near the Achilles tendon. * It shares its duty as the Stream point of the Kidney channel also.

K. Channel Base Point: *Kidney 3* *Mula Vrikka Sira*

KAPHA (PM)

The Pericardium channel Base Point

The Pericardium channel's Base point is at the wrist crease, * sharing its function as the Stream point of the Pericardium channel.

P. Channel Base Point: *Pericardium 7* *Mula Talahridaya Sira*

The Tridosha channel Base Point

The 3D channel has its Base point at the wrist, back of the arm.

3D Channel Base Point: *Tridosha 4* *Mula Tridosha Sira*

PITTA (AM)

The Gall Bladder channel Base Point

The Gallbladder's Base point is on the outside area of the instep of the foot.

GB. Channel Base Point: *Gallbladder 40* *Mula Pittashaya Sira*

The Liver channel Base Point

The Liver has its Base point on the foot, near the large toe. * This point is also the Stream point of the Liver channel

Lv Channel Base Point: *Liver 3 Mula Yakrit Sira*

The cleft points

The Cleft Points (Antara Siras)

Each of the twelve organ channels has a cleft point, *Antara sira*. Antara means a cleft or crevice. This is where *Prana* is deeply retained along a channel and allowing the energy to supplement the channel's energy.

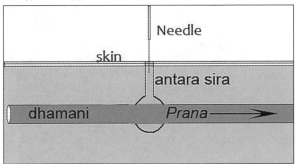

***Fig.19.** Cleft point*

Cleft points assist in treating *acute* diseases and pain of the related organs, their channels and the areas they cross.

L.6. (CLEFT POINT)

The Lung channel has its Cleft point on the radial side

of inside of arm, 5 angulis distal to elbow crease.

Lung Channel Cleft Point L.6 *Antara Phuphusa Sira*

LI.7. (CLEFT POINT)

The Large Intestine channel has its Cleft point about 5 angulis from wrist crease, on radial side of back of hand.

LI Channel Cleft Point LI7 *Antara Sthulantra Sira*

St.34. (CLEFT POINT)

The Stomach channel has its Cleft point in the depression 2 angulis above kneecap and to the lateral aspect of thigh.

Stomach Channel Cleft Point St34 *Antara Amashaya Sira*

Sp.8 (CLEFT POINT)

The Spleen channel has its Cleft point 3 angulis below the tibial protrusion at medial aspect of knee.

Spleen Channel Cleft Point Sp8 *Antara Pliha Sira*

H.6 (CLEFT POINT)

The Heart channel has its Cleft point half anguli above wrist crease on radial side of arm.

Heart Channel Cleft Point H6 *Antara Hridaya Sira*

SI.6. (CLEFT POINT)

The Small Intestine channel has its Cleft point in the depression, at distal joint of ulna/radial bones, back of hand.

Small Intestine Channel Cleft Point SI6 *Antara Grahani Sira*

UB.63. (CLEFT POINT)

The Small Intestine channel has its Cleft point in the depression, below malleolus and frontal to it (about 1.5 angulis).

Urinary Bladder Channel Cleft Point UB63 *Antara Mutrashaya Sira*

K.5 (CLEFT POINT)

The Kidney channel has its Cleft point below and rear to internal malleolus

Kidney Channel Cleft Point K5 *Antara Vrikka Sira*

P.4 (CLEFT POINT)

The Pericardium channel has its Cleft point 5 angulis above the crease of the wrist, in medial aspect of arm, between the two tendons.

Pericardium Channel Cleft Point P4 *Antara Manodhara Sira*

3D.7. (CLEFT POINT)

The Tridosha channel has its Cleft point in the depression, 3 angulis above wrist crease, on back of arm.

Tridosha Channel Cleft Point 3D7 *Antara Dosha Sira*

GB.36. (CLEFT POINT)

The Gallbladder channel has its Cleft point 7 angulis above the external malleolus, near the front edge of fibula.

Gallbladder Channel Cleft Point GB36 *Antara Pittashaya Sira*

Lv.6 (CLEFT POINT)

The Liver channel has its Cleft point 7 angulis from the internal malleolus, directly above it.

Liver Channel Cleft Point Lv6 *Antara Yakrit Sira*

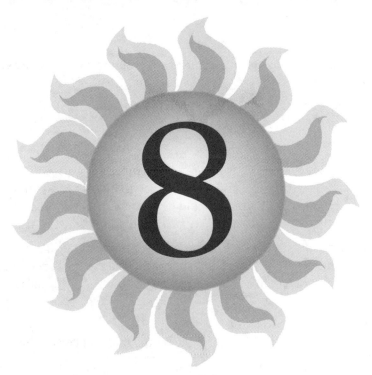

Techniques and treatment

Needling Effects

Needles

An acupuncture needle is called a *suchi* in marmapuncture. The materials (needles, etc.) used for needling have their own qualities and effects on the doshas, so consequently attention should be paid if gold, silver or other materials are used for needles. For instance, silver needles may aggravate Vata or Kapha on a subtle level or when dealing with emotional or psychological issues due to its sedating/cold effect and when used excessively. Gold may aggravate Pitta, due to its stimulating/heating effects, yet the correct material for the person's bodytype will enhance the therapeutic effect of needling.

Today, we tend to use needles made of stainless steel, which consists of various metals and is usually considered as having a neutral energetic effect in comparison to gold or silver.

The needle consists of the blade which is used to puncture. Its length can vary but the usual length we use today tends to be 25mm. The gauge can also vary but we tend to use finer needles, of 0.22mm gauge. This is in keeping with the general rule of not trying to aggravate Vata by perhaps using needles or depths which can cause pain or major discomfort.

A needle may also consist of a handle which allows grip while performing insertion and when removing the needle from the patient's body.

The thickness of the needle is carefully mentioned by Sushruta as explained by Ranade *et al.*

> *"Sushruta in Sharira sthana 8 'Siravyadha' has advised puncturing the channels (sira) by using needles, which are as small as 'vrihi' (vrihi is the outer cover of the rice grain which is pointed at both ends). This means that the acupuncture needle should be as pointed as vrihi. Needles now available of this caliber are of no 26."* [103]

Generally a quality needle such as the brand Seirin made in Japan is preferable because of the excellent quality and sharpness, but some of the Chinese made needles are also acceptable. For puncturing of the ear a shorter needle of 13 mm can be used.

Needles are kept inserted in the body for a period of time according to the client's bodytype, with Vata clients requiring less time than Pitta or Kapha, in general.

The needle manipulation depends greatly on the dosha being treated as certain actions may aggravate a particular dosha. Excessive hand manipulation of a needle may aggravate Vata but may indeed strengthen Kapha. As with marma massage, in marmapuncture we rotate the needle (once inserted in marma or sira) clockwise to sedate the flow of prana and anticlockwise to stimulate the flow. However this may not always be necessary or desirable as allowing the needle in situ to stimulate the body may cause it to find its own balance in the flow of prana.

Usual marmapuncture treatment may take up to an hour, the length of time depending on the bodytype or constitution of the client. These effects will be clearly noticed in clinical practice.

Needling Effects According to Doshas

REQUIREMENT	DOSHA
Marma Depth of Insertion	
Shallow	Vata
Medium	Pitta
Deeper	Kapha
Number of Needles	
Minimum	Vata

---

103 Drs. Subhash Ranade, Avinash Lele and David Frawley. *Secrets of Marma.* International Academy of Ayurveda Publishing, Pune, India. (pg. 98).

Medium	Pitta
Most (a maximum of 15 needles)	Kapha
Needle Material	
Gold or Silver (with care)	Vata
Silver	Pitta
Gold	Kapha
Needling Action/Insertion	
Gentle, rhythmic	Vata
Medium rhythmic	Pitta
Intense, fast, erratic (with care)	Kapha
Needling Time	
15-30 minutes	Vata
20-40 minutes	Pitta
40-60 minutes	Kapha
Electric Pulse	
Slow, rhythmic, less intense	Vata
Medium, regular, rhythmic	Pitta
Intense, fast, erratic (with care)	Kapha
Agni-karma (Heat Application, with or without needles)	
May require heat but not excessively (may over stimulate Vata)	Vata
Does not generally require heat	Pitta
May require heat	Kapha

Needle Insertion

Depth of Insertion

When the needle is inserted at the appropriate sira, care should be taken of the underlying structures so as not to create a medical emergency such as in the sira L1 (Apalapa marma). This location is directly over the lung and deep insertion may actually puncture the lung and cause it to collapse. So needling here is best avoided by the novice. Depth of insertion depends on the general anatomical locations.

The general guideline is for muscular areas (e.g. thighs) the depth is up to 5mm, while for other areas the depth is about 2.5mm. (Sushruta Sharira, 8/9). In practice though, these measurement can be exceeded with caution.

Each sira has its own depth of insertion listed in the Siras section of this book. Nevertheless, Ayurvedic acupuncture does not necessarily require very deep insertion, as it may occur in other systems of acupuncture.

When the prana flowing through the dhamani and into the sira comes in contact with the needle (*suchi*) at the appropriate depth, a sensation of tightness will often be felt on the needle. This is called *suchigraha*, meaning 'seizing of the needle'. It indicates that the needle is placed at the right angle and correct depth and it should now be left there for the appropriate length of time.

Sometimes, it may be somewhat difficult to remove the needle before its appropriate time but when the body is ready to release it, the needle will easily be removed.

Angle of Insertion

Sushruta has advised insertion at some siras in a (a) Perpendicular direction, (b) Horizontal direction or in an (c) Oblique direction to the skin (Sushruta Sutra, 5/4).

Examples of the oblique insertion is that of needling points on the eyebrows. Horizontal insertion includes needling of the sira related to Sthapani marma (G24.5).

Perpendicular insertion is that of the St36 (Earth) Samudra Sira.

In addition, it will generally be noticed that needles may sometimes lean towards or against the direction of pranic flow through the particular dhamani where the sira is embedded. We can often use this as a technique for increasing or reducing energy in the dhamani.

Locating Marmas/ Siras

It is therefore sometimes easy to locate a marma or a sira, as it is either sensitive to pressure (e.g. L.I.4) or else forms a slightly hollow area on the body (e.g. H7, L9 etc.).

Marmas can also be located by a measurement. This is a 'finger measurement' or *Anguli*. A *marma* may be located thus, e.g. *two anguli from the wrist crease, for Pericardium 6.* Thus the measurement of anguli is relative to the patient and not the therapist.

Another way of determining an anguli is the measurement across the width of the base of the fingers (without thumb) and divide this measurement by eight. For instance, a width of 9cm means that the person's anguli would be 1.125 cms.

The length of the middle finger between the two creases when the finger is bent (of the patient and not of the practitioner) is usually taken as one anguli as is the width of the thumb. An *angulometer* is a device used for measuring angulis.

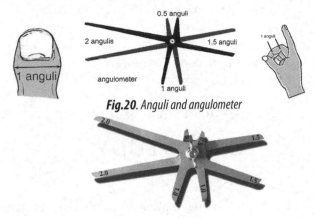

***Fig.20.** Anguli and angulometer*

The above angulometer was originally conceived by the doctors in Sri Lanka, under the auspices of the late Prof. Dr. A. Jayasuriya. The above design is by the author.

Marmapuncture Treatment

Based upon a thorough Ayurvedic diagnosis, the treatment can then proceed. The diagnosis may include tongue, pulse or nail diagnoses and may also include palpation of certain siras.

Treatment may need to take into account srotas or physiological channels which may be affected by the imbalance, the dhatus or tissues involved, the sub-doshas that may be helpful and lastly the organs involved in the dis-ease process.

Within this scheme a sira may also be chosen to provide relaxation for the patient, another to increase agni or metabolic fire or yet another sira to strengthen Ojas or immune essence of the body. Sometimes, some siras/marmas have multi-effects and so, one sira can be used for several effects.

Point Combination

Selection of siras or acupoints for a particular treatment is not unlike selection of various herbs to form a balanced Ayurvedic formula. Combination of points which are relevant to the presenting condition most often provides a positive treatment for the patient, however masterly selection of points which comes with experience may often provide a better or more specific response. The master marmapuncturist utilizes the least number of needles to achieve the best possible outcome.

Sterility

Sterilization of equipment to be utilized is essential. Nowadays needles can be purchased which are disposable. Insertion and removal of needles will need to be performed carefully. Also, care should be exercised in ensuring all needles utilized are accounted for and have been disposed of appropriately in a sharps disposal container. It is often recommended to swab the treated location with an alcohol swap to prevent infection. The local Health and Safety regulations for piercing the body should be followed.

Typical Case Studies

CASE STUDY 1

CLIENT:

Male, thirty years old, professional martial artist (3rd degree black belt).

CLIENT HISTORY

Although the client did not suffer from any particular ailments and appeared very physically fit, he attended the clinic as a preparation for an important upcoming national martial arts competition. He had heard from friends that the marmapuncture treatment could help him to better focus and remain calm.

AYURVEDIC DIAGNOSIS

The client was of a pitta constitution (although there was a certain amount of kapha e.g. muscles). Lack of chest body hair indicated pitta as did his radial pulses, especially strong in the pitta/ liver-gallbladder position. His pitta prakruti was also demonstrated on the tongue with very little or no white tongue coating (nirama).

Trigunas

His strong desire to be involved in competitions and to win indicated that his Rajas was strong.

Tridoshas

Pitta needed to be balanced (otherwise there may be anger which may be counterproductive) in order to keep a calm mind during the match. Some of the subdoshas would also be treated.

The Five Elements (pancha-mahabhutas)

Wind needed to be kept in check (nervousness) and Earth supported for grounding.

AYURVEDIC ACUPUNCTURE TREATMENT

TREATMENT PLAN
Treatment involved allowing prana to flow unimpeded throughout the body and we suggested treatment based on pranic balancing (Akashic balancing). Impedance in the body at any location (e.g. the liver) may cause friction, inflammation and blockages. The points chosen would be principal prana sub-doshic points or siras, some of which are also major marmas and which may also involve the chakras. A number of other supporting points would also be added in this case. Sensory stimuli such as music and incense were also used in keeping with Akashic balancing principles and the client's own constitution.

POINT SELECTION
Nervous System/Manovaha srotas: G20 – Adhipati marma, Crown chakra. Adhipati - the 'Over Lord' of all marmas and siras, balances pranic energy and treats the nervous system. Also works on the psychological level and the mind, manas- helps connect mind and heart. H7 – Hridaya Sira (Earth point)- relaxes heart, nerves and calms vata.

PranaVayu: Pe8, K1, Talahridaya marmas. Pe8 Fire point to balance mental Tejas.

Vyana Vayu: C17 (Hridaya marma) – treats the breasts, circulates Prana (Vyana vayu), and also rakta vaha srotas.

Apana Vayu: Sp6 was used in this case, Apana vayu sira - balances downward flow, homeostatic, immune, treats kidney, liver and spleen.

Udana Vayu: Pe6 (Antara sira). Udana vayu – subtle flow (thoughts, emotions).

Samana Vayu: SI5 Fire point (treats Samana vayu).

OTHER POINTS:
3D9 (Indrabasti marma). This point assists metabolism.

Lv2 (Pada Kshipra marma –Sara yakrt sira). Bhuta Agni – Fire point controls Wind (Wheel of Control)

G24.5 (Sthapani marma) Brow chakra. Pituitary and mental support. Ojas and endocrine system. Balances mind and nervous system.

Homeostatic Points:

St36 (Samudra amashaya sira) Earth point.

LI11 (Kurpara marma [Samudra sthulantra sira]) point to strengthen the immune system.

RESULTS

After the initial treatment, the client felt extremely relaxed and light. A few minutes later he felt energetic and motivated and there was no pain or any symptom demonstrated. Client was advised to drink water in order to assist detox and to ensure hydration, (this is especially important in Akashic balancing). The client left the clinic after an appropriate amount of time and was due to fly to the national competition on the weekend, two days later.

The client returned to the clinic seven days after the competition. He mentioned he had felt well all the time but what was surprising for him was the fact that not only had he won the national championship (although he had won other competitions before) but commented on how focused he had been, was able to easily counter his opponent's attacks and then defeat him. Althroughout, he felt calm and with no feeling of anger at all.

He has since undertaken meditation, especially chakra meditation and has concentrated on instructing others in the martial arts. His all-consuming desire to compete is now more balanced and he is undergoing further rank training, currently going for his fourth black belt (attainment of knowledge- sattva). He now reports to the clinic every three months for what he calls a 'tune-up' and seems settled and positive. He was recently awarded his fourth black belt.

CASE STUDY 2

CLIENT:
Female, in her late forties.

CLIENT HISTORY
The client attended the clinic reporting of lower back pain which she had suffered for a few weeks.

AYURVEDIC DIAGNOSIS
The client appeared to be of a vata/ pitta prakruti with vata nerves.

The area of complaint on the rear torso was in the lower back, directly involving around the kidneys/urinary bladder/ large intestines which are in the vata area. Pulse also demonstrated some liver imbalance which could cause her some hypertension, of which she was aware.

AYURVEDIC ACUPUNCTURE TREATMENT

TREATMENT PLAN

Tridoshas
The treatment would involve calming down vata and supporting or balancing pitta in the liver. Utilize points that balance the vata area.

POINTS USED:
Nervous System/Manovaha srotas: G20 – Adhipati marma, H7 – Hridaya sira.

Base or Root point of Vata: LI4 (Kshipra marma).

Metabolism: UB57, 3D9, Annavaha srotas, Indrabasti marmas, lumbago.

Support of lower back/Vata: UB40 Ambhu vaha srotas (water flow, urinary system), sciatica.

Apana vayu: Sp6.

OTHER POINTS:
Lv2 (Pada Kshipra marma –Sara yakrt sira). Bhuta Agni – Fire point controls wind (Wheel of Control).

G24.5 (Sthapani marma), Ojas.

Lv 3 (Kurccha marma) treatment for hypertension (with care).

RESULTS

After treatment, the client reported less pain in lower back and a relaxed feeling in both legs. She also felt relaxed.

The second treatment was given a week later, the client had felt less pain in the lower back and so a similar treatment was given.

At the third treatment, the client reported that after feeling some pain during the week she decided to take a strong pain killer but this appeared to have had a negative effect on her by raising her blood pressure significantly. After taking her blood pressure it was obvious that it was very high. Lv3 was included in the treatment which did lower the blood pressure to an acceptable level.

The client had several other treatments and the lower back pain had subsequently stopped and had not returned. Her blood pressure is now normal.

CASE STUDY 3

CLIENT:
Female, aged 45.

CLIENT HISTORY:
The client suffered from migraines and constipation.

DIAGNOSIS:
The client was of kapha prakruti, poor circulation, low Agni and slow metabolism. Pulse was kapha, slow and even. Tongue was of kapha shape with some ama. Migraine was Common migraine with forehead pain (kapha).

AYURVEDIC ACUPUNCTURE TREATMENT

TREATMENT PLAN
Treatment involved improving metabolism and circulation as well as elimination.

POINTS USED:
G20- (Adhipati marma). To relax the client.

To stimulate Agni:

3D 9 (Hasta Indrabasti marma).

UB57 (Pada Indrabasti marma).

SI 5 River (Fire) point of small intestine.

To balance Gallbladder function:

GB 40 Base point of Gallbladder.

Lv 5 Bridge point of Liver.

To improve pranic and bodily flow in torso (Tridosha):

3D 10 Sea (Earth) point of the Tridosha channel.

3D 4 Base of the Tridosha channel.

OTHER POINTS:
Sp6 (Apana vayu) to assist elimination (urinary bladder, bowels, etc).

LI 5 River (Fire) point of large intestine to strengthen agni in bowels.

K 5 Cleft (Antara sira) point of Kidney channel.

RESULTS

After two treatments, the client reported her bowel action had improved and had become regular. Her migraines had reduced in frequency and strength and she felt more relaxed.

Next visit, the client reported she had been angry, so liver and gall bladder points were used to stabilize these. Additional points used were Lv3, GB40 and Sthapani marma or G24.5 which affects the pituitary gland (master hormonal gland) and the Brow chakra. The treatment was effective and the client did not experience any further migraines nor was she angry for a period of a month. After a mild migraine, the client returned and several further treatments were performed with no constipation or migraines occurring.

At a follow up treatment a month later, the client reported no constipation or migraine problems, she's now calmer and has lost some weight.

Marmapuncture
treatment of common diseases

Most diseases can be differentiated by their presenting symptoms due to one of the three doshas being vitiated. Consequently disease treatment relies on a thorough Tridosha differentiation and then selection of the appropriate herb(s) or sira(s) which can rebalance said imbalance. Usually a formula of points and herbs is selected for its overall treatment of the disease.

An example of such Ayurvedic formula is *Chyavan prash* which can contain between 20 to 60 herbs in its preparation (depending on manufacturer) but most formulas contain fewer herbs. For example *Hingashtak* with ten ingredients or herbs (such as Caraway, Asafetida etc).

Likewise most marmapuncture point formulas have fewer than 15 points which are treated by filiform needles.

There is an ancient saying that "an extrovert practitioner will utilize many needles while the master will carefully choose a handful."

(VPK) means **V**ata**P**itta**K**apha while - or + means it reduces or increases a dosha. For example (VP-K+) means the herb reduces Vata and Pitta and increases Kapha. On the other hand, = means that the herb is balanced for all three doshas (e.g. VPK=).

The following disease treatments are basic but functional, as generally a full Ayurvedic diagnosis is required and may involve choosing points and other herbs based on the individual diagnosis which is much more comprehensive. The clinical case studies shown in the previous chapter 8 are clear examples which demonstrate this formulation.

1. Anemia
Anemia is characterized by the absence of RBCs and hemoglobin (iron transport protein). It tends to reflect an iron deficiency and thus related to *Vata* vitiation. Ayurveda calls this disease '*Pandu Roga*' (pale disease).

Symptoms include paleness of the skin, especially of the conjunctiva and edges of the tongue. There may also be hypotension, asthenia, dyspnea, dizziness and weak, rapid pulse. All of these point to *Vata* disorders.

Herbal therapy
Ayurvedic treatment for anemia may include Yellow dock herb (PK-V+) which can be used to supplement iron and is useful for Pitta type anemia but should not be used in high Vata emaciation. *Chyavan prash* jelly may assist in anemia. *Ashwagandha* (VK-P+) and *Bhringaraj* (VPK=) can also be useful in anemia as can *Punarnava* (PK-V+) and *Manjishta* (PK-V+).

Marmapuncture

Sira	Indication
L 7	Dizziness
LI 11	Sea point influences *Vata* and large intestine.
P 6	Bridge point, affects and relieves the chest area (shallow breathing).
UB 18	Liver rear organ point.
UB 19	Gallbladder rear organ point.
St 36	Sea point affects the stomach, increasing the strength of the element of Earth in the body (decreases *Vata*).
Sp 6	*Apana Vayu sira*, meeting point of the three solid organ channels of the lower limbs, which influences the lower trunk area (*Vata*).

2. Asthma
Asthma involves, difficulty in breathing, wheezing, chest tightness and stiffness. In Ayurveda it is called *Tomaka Shvasa*. Asthma attacks caused by allergens can relate to immune system deficiencies. Ayurveda holds that asthma imbalances originate in the digestive system (especially *Agni* disturbances). Correct diag-

nosis is essential to understand which *Dosha* is affected. The type of asthma related to *Vata* is characterized by dyspnea and cough (which is also related to stress). The *Kapha* type is related to congestion and mucus, while a rapid pulse, bounding, with a thick yellow coating corresponds to a *Pitta* imbalance.

For *Vata* type asthma means puncturing points of the lung and large intestine channels. This is intended to eliminate cold and Wind.

Pitta type asthma is treated by needling of the Sea Point of the lung channel (L 5) to increase Water and decrease Fire (according to the wheel of control), since water controls fire.

The *Kapha* type includes needling of Stomach 40 *sira* to relax the chest and remove phlegm. This point of the Stomach channel is related to the Earth element. Consequently, Earth puncturing points (St 36 and L 9) of the organs related to the element Air (Lung and Large intestine) can be tonified according to parent and child rule and the wheel of support.

Herbal therapy

Ayurvedic treatment for asthma may include *Trikatu* (for Vata and Kapha) and *Gotu kola* (for Pitta). Cardamon (VK-P+), Flaxseed (V-PK+) and Mullein (PK-V+).

Marmapuncture

Sira   **Indication**

Vata

UB 13   Rear Lung organ point. Balances the lung.

L 7   Bridge point between the channels of the lung and large intestine. Useful to treat imbalances of both channels, reduces cold and wind.

LI 4   Base point of the Large Intestine channel. It is prescribed for the same I imbalances (*Vata's* primary site organ).

Pitta

St 40   Bridge point between the Stomach and Spleen channels. Asthma point, removes phlegm and reduces heat in the lung.

L 5   Sea point (Water). Balances the lung and reduces heat.

Kapha

St 40   Bridge Point between the Stomach and Spleen channels. Asthma point, removes phlegm from lung.

3. Amenorrhea

This imbalance is characterized by the absence of menstruation. *Siras* are selected from channels found in the *Vata* area of the torso and lower limbs or organs positioned in the pelvis (reproductive organs).

Herbal therapy

Ayurvedic treatment for amenorrhea may include *Kumari* or Aloe (VPK=), Pennyroyal (VK-P+), *Shatapatri* or Rose Flowers (VPK=), *Tila* or Sesame seeds (V-PK+), *Haridra* or Turmeric (K-PV+) and *Manjishta* (PK-V+).

Marmapuncture

Sira	Indication
UB 32	Removes stagnant blood in the uterus.
St 29	Indicated in amenorrhea, removes blood congestion.
LI 4	Base Point of the Large Intestine channel (*Vata*) which affects the pelvis.
Sp 6	Meeting point of the Liver, Spleen and Kidney channels. Regulates blood flow to the reproductive system.
Lv 2	Spring point, regulates the entry and exit of blood from the liver.
Sp 10	It affects blood circulation and promotes menstrual bleeding.
UB 18	Liver rear organ point. Affects the liver blood flow.
UB 20	Spleen rear organ point, which regulates Spleen.
UB 23	Kidney rear organ point. Kidney affects Vata and the reproductive organs.
St 25	Large intestine front organ point.
St 36	Stomach Sea Point.

4. Common cold

The common cold can be caused by four different types of imbalances, but essentially is caused by deficiencies in the immune system and is characterized by a set of physical symptoms whose primary function is to remove toxins. The accumulation or aggravation of the three doshas during a particular season and the incorrect resolution in the subsequent season may lead to colds. The imbalance of the three doshas (Tridoshas) can lead to chronic cold.

Herbal therapy

Ayurvedic treatment for the common cold may include herbs like Ginger (VK-P+), Cinnamon (VK-P+), *Katphala* or Bayberry (VK-P+), *Gandana* or Yarrow (PK-V+) and *Pippali* or Indian Long Pepper (VK-P+).

Marmapuncture

Sira	Indication
Vata	(Dark grey coating, pale tongue)

UB 12   Reduces **Vata** and Wind, relieves headaches.

LI 20   Decreases Wind pathogenic factor in the head.

LI 4   Base Point of the Large Intestine (*Vata*), improves colds.

L 7   Bridge point between the channels of the lung and large intestine. Improves nasal congestion, headache and cough.

Pitta   (Yellow tongue coating, red tongue body)

GB 20   Febrile illnesses, colds, headaches and symptoms of *Pitta* in the head and neck.

3D 5   Febrile illnesses, headaches.

Kapha   (Whitish tongue coating)

LI 4   Base Point of the Large Intestine (*Vata*), increases heat and decreases cold.

K 7   River Point, increases fire by supporting the Ether element.

5. Dysmenorrhea

Dysmenorrhea (*Rakta Pradara*) is a disorder of the female reproductive system, and can be divided into two types: (a) Menorrhagia, characterized by excessive bleeding during the menstrual cycle, and (b) Metrorrhagia, including excessive menstruation intervals irregular. This is usually caused by Pitta imbalances that affect the hormonal system. When Pitta is out of balance, bleeding can occur anywhere in the body, such as the nose, rectum, etc.

Herbal therapy

Ayurvedic treatment for dysmenorrhea may include herbs like Asafetida (VK-P+), Nutmeg (VK-P+), *Jatamansi* and Cyperus. For Pitta, nervine herbs such as Passionflower (PK-V+), Hops (PK-V+), and Skullcap (PK-Vo) are also appropriate.

Marmapuncture

Sira	Indication
Sp 10	This *sira* activates corrects blood circulation.
Sp 8	Used to improve menstrual cramps and pain.
LI 4	Used for pain relief during menstruation.

St 27	Removes stagnant blood in the uterus and improves symptoms of pain in the reproductive system.
UB 20-UB 23	Regulate the spleen and kidney organs, source of blood formation.
Sp 6	Sea point. Strengthens spleen function (blood supply).
St 36	Sea point, strengthens stomach function (blood formation source).
UB 40	Sea point, removes excess heat in the blood.

6. Dysentery

Dysentery can be caused by parasites like amoebas (*Pravahika*) involving *Kapha*, or of bacterial origin (*Raktatisa*), involving Pitta.

Herbal therapy

Ayurvedic treatment may include herbs like *Shatavari* (PV-K+), Raspberry (PK-V+), *Bala* (VPK=), and Fenugreek (VK-P+).

Marmapuncture

Sira **Indication**

Kapha

UB 20	Spleen rear organ point, indicated in dysentery disorders, as it increases warmth in the spleen and removes intestinal congestion.
UB 21	Stomach rear organ point, indicated in dysentery, it warms the stomach.
Sp 6	Assists in the removal of moisture and dampness (*Kapha*) and strengthens the role of the spleen (*Kapha* organ).
St 36	Eliminates intestinal congestion.

Pitta

St 44	Spring point (Water), removes heat.
LI 11	Sea *Sira* (Earth), child of fire, removes heat especially in the large intestine.
Sp 9	Sea *Sira* (Water), controls fire, by strengthening the Spleen.
St 25	Large Intestine organ *Sira*, indicated in dysentery by reducing LI organ congestion.
St 37	Sea point of the LI in the leg, removes congestion in the LI organ.
LI 4	Base point of the large intestine (*Vata*), indicated in dysentery and Intestine syndromes. Removes organ congestion.

7. Diarrhea

It can be caused by the imbalance of (1) *Vata* and fear (2) *Pitta* (3) *Kapha* (4) the 3D. (5) Ama. The best way to treat *Ama* is by using herbs with bitter and pungent tastes. Bitter herbs tend to release toxins (*Ama*) from the tissues, while pungent destroys it (ama). Besides puncturing of *siras*, diarrhea can be treated by drinking boiled rice water (with a pinch of salt to taste), this serves to decrease diarrhea and is very useful for chronic cases.

Herbal therapy

Ayurvedic treatment for diarrhea may include herbs like *Bibhitaki* (KP-V+), *Haritaki* (VPK=), *Padma* or Lotus (PV-K+) and Pomegranate (PK-Vo).

Marmapuncture

Sira   Indication

St 25   LI organ point in Stomach channel. Regulates LI proper organ function.

UB 25   Large Intestine rear organ point. It also regulates transportation in the large intestine, in addition of treating diarrhea.

St 36   Sea point, strengthens transportation in the Spleen and Stomach (*Kapha*).

UB 23   Kidney rear organ point. It balances Kidney and supports *Vata* area in the torso.

K 3   Stream *Sira* (Earth). The Earth element (Parent) supports the Air/Wind and large intestine (Child).

8. Erysipelas

Erysipelas can be caused by imbalances in: 1) *Vata* 2) *Pitta* 3) *Kapha* 4) 3D and 5) Trauma.

Herbal therapy

Ayurvedic treatment for erysipelas may include an herb like Burdock (PK-V+).

Marmapuncture

Sira   Indication

UB 40   Sea *Sira* (Earth). Removes heat from the blood to act as child dissipating energy from parent (Fire - UB 60)

P 3   Sea *Sira* (Water). Removing heat from the blood by encouraging Water.

LI 11   Sea *Sira* (Earth), child of Fire, removes heat especially in the large intestine.

LI 4   Base *Sira* of the large intestine (*Vata*), removes heat from the Intestines. Removes LI organ congestion.

9. Hiccup

Hiccup or *Hikka Roga* is caused by the vitiation of *Vata*, Vayu or Wind/Air which in this case tends to rise and cause hiccups.

Herbal therapy

Ayurvedic treatment for hiccup may include an herb like *Lavanga* or Cloves (KV-P+).

Marmapuncture

Sira   Indication

UB 17   Stabilizes ascending Wind *Vata*.

P 6   *Udana Vayu Sira*, Bridge point, affects and diminishes fullness in the chest area.

St 36   Sea point (Earth). Indicated in stomach syndromes, which is affected by the rising *Vata*.

10. Hysteria

Hysteria is usually related to *Vata*, the subtlest of humors, which is also related to the nervous system.

Herbal therapy

Ayurvedic treatment for hysteria may include herbs like *Aluka* or Wild Yam (VP-K+), *Hingu* or Asafetida (VK-P+), *Nagakeshara* or Saffron (VPK=). *Nagadamani* or Mugwort (VK-P+) and Pennyroyal (VK-P+).

Marmapuncture

Sira   Indication

LI 4   Base Point of the large intestine (*Vata*) which affects the pelvis.

Lv 3   Stream Point adjusts liver function and helps reduce convulsions.

K 1   Well Sira (Ether). Subtly affects Vata and improves unconsciousness.

P 6   Bridge point, decreases feelings of suffocation.

H 7   Stream point (Earth), *Hridaya sira*. Indicated in Hysteria.

11. Haemorrhoids

Hemorrhoids (*Arsha*) are varicosities of the veins in the rectal area caused by congestion in the large intestine. They can also cause much pain and bleeding.

When accompanied by heat and humidity they are related to *Pitta*, more painful when dry they are then related to *Vata*, and those associated with congestion and cold associated to *Kapha*.

Herbal therapy
Ayurvedic treatment for hemorrhoids may include herbs like *Guggulu* or Guggul-Indian Bedellium (KV-P+), *Gokshura* or Caltrops (VPK=), *Amalaki* or Emblic myrobalan (PV-K+) and *Amla vetasa* or Yellow Dock (PK-V+).

Marmapuncture
Sira   Indication

UB 57   Indicated in hemorrhoidal syndromes.

UB 32   Indicated in pain of the lower back and lower limb.

G1   Point of the perineum, it is indicated for treatment of hemorrhoids due to the proximity of the location to the rectum.

12. Hypertension
The excessive rise in blood pressure is known in Ayurveda as *Rakta Vata* (hypertension). This stems from the imbalance of *Vata*, which occurs as a result of rigidity, narrowing and tension of the arteries (*Vata* can remove moisture from the blood due to its drying qualities). *Rakta Vata* means "*Vata* in Blood".

Herbal therapy
Ayurvedic treatment hypertension may include herbs like Skullcap (PK- V+), Hawthorn berries (V-PK+), *Rashona* or Garlic (VK-P+) and Burdock (PK-V+).

Marmapuncture
Sira   Indication

LI 11   Sea point (Earth). Treats Wind/Air in the large intestine and balances *Vata*.

St 36   Sea point (Earth). It is related to the Earth, parent of the Air element, so that it tonifies *Vata*.

GB 20   Indicated in vertigo and headache caused by hypertension.

Lv 3   Stream Point (Earth), tonifying Wind/Air and *Vata*. Indicated in dizziness and headaches.

Sp 9   Sea *Sira* (Water). It is a Water point, so it treats *Vata* by supporting the kidneys.

13. Impotence

Impotence (*Klavya*) can be caused by following imbalances: 1) *Vata*, 2) *Pitta*, 3) *Kapha*, 4) the three *doshas*. Usually related to kidney imbalance or *Vata*.

Herbal therapy

Ayurvedic treatment for impotence may include herbs like *Aluka* or Wild Yam (VP-K+), *Padma* or Lotus (PV-K+) and *Gokshura* or Caltrops (VPK=) which can also increase semen.

Marmapuncture

Sira   **Indication**

Vata

UB 15   Heart rear organ point. Balances and relaxes the nervous system so it calms *Vata*.

Pitta

H 7   Stream Point of the Heart, is related to Earth, child of fire.

H 8   Removes sedate the point heat source.

Kapha

Sp 6   This point (*Apana sira*) is the conjunction of the meridians of spleen, liver and kidney, which are important because they go through the genital and *Vata* area.

General

UB25   Large Intestine rear organ point, corrects *Vata* by treating the large intestine.

K 3   Stream sira (Earth). Strengthen *Vata* and large intestine according to the parent-child rule.

14. Jaundice

Jaundice (*Kamala*), is usually caused by inflammation of the liver and if when examination of the tongue a yellowish coating is present, this is due to the imbalance relating to *Pitta*. On the other hand if the coating is whitish, this is caused by the imbalance of *Kapha* affecting the liver.

Herbal therapy

Ayurvedic treatment for jaundice may include herbs like *Nimba* or Neem (PK-V+), *Manjishta* or Indian Madder (PK-V+), *Amla-vetasa* or Rhubarb (PK-V+), *Kirata* or Gentian (PK-V+) and Dandelion (PK-V+).

Marmapuncture

Sira   Indication

Kapha

Sp 9   Sea *Sira* (Water). Reduces phlegm in *Kapha* syndromes.

St 36   Sea *Sira* (Earth). Supports the stomach in *Kapha* syndromes.

Pitta

GB 34   Sea *Sira* (Earth). Reduces heat or *Pitta* by acting as the child of fire (GB 38). Affects the liver, as the gallbladder is associated with it internally.

Lv 3   Base and Stream Point (Earth). Reduces liver heat or *Pitta* by acting as the child of Fire (Lv2).

UB 48   Indicated in jaundice.

GB 24   Gallbladder front organ *Sira*. Useful for treating gallbladder syndromes, including jaundice.

15. Leucorrhea

Leucorrhoea (*Shweta Pradara*), is characterized by a whitish vaginal discharge, usually caused by *Kapha* imbalance affecting the reproductive system, especially common in women of *Vata* constitution. When the flow is more abundant and yellowish, the gallbladder and liver are affected.

Herbal therapy

Ayurvedic treatment for leucorrhea may include herbs like *Shatavari* or Asparagus racemosus (PV-K+), *Haritaki* or Terminalia chebula (VPK=), *Guggulu* or Guggul resin (KV-P+), Bala or Indian country mallow (VPK= but K+ in excess) and *Dadima* or Pomegranate (generally VPK=).

Marmapuncture

Sira   Indication

UB 23   Kidney rear organ point. Tonifies Prana, especially in the kidneys (which affect the reproductive system).

UB 32   Indicated in Leucorrhoea as it is in the Vata area of the unbalance in the channel.

UB 30   Similar to above.

Lv 5   Bridge Point. Reduces Fire- heat and brings balance to the gallbladder and liver.

Sp 9   Sea *Sira* (Water). This point when tonified, strengthens spleen function, reducing heat.

16. Hypotension

The reduction of normal blood pressure is called *Nyuna Raktachapa*, hypotension is an imbalance that is related to *Vata*, affecting mostly people of *Vata* constitution.

Herbal therapy

Ayurvedic treatment for hypotension may include herbs like *Lavanga* or Cloves and *Yashti madu* or Licorice root (VP-K+).

Marmapuncture

Sira	Indication
Lv 3	Stream Point (Earth). As parent of Wind, the Lv3 tonifies and increases the correct Prana level in the large intestine, which raises blood pressure.
P 6	Bridge Point of Pericardium (and 3D channels), affects the flow of body fluids through the body, improves circulation and blood pressure.

17. Mumps

Mumps (*Karnamulaka*) is generally caused by imbalances or infections related to *Pitta*. They are characterized by inflammation and swelling of the parotid gland. The heat affects the *3D* and large intestine meridians which cross the area of inflammation.

Herbal therapy

Ayurvedic treatment for mumps may include an herb like Mullein (PK-V+).

Marmapuncture

Sira	Indication
LI 4	Base point of the large intestine (*Vata*). Indicated for facial swelling, decreasing the heat on the meridian of the LI and face area.
LI 11	Sea point (Earth). Drain the heat of fire element, as it is the child in a mother-child rule and removes heat from the LI.
3D 17	Located in the area, improving the swelling and pain.
St 6	Similar to above.

18. Pneumonia

Pneumonia (*Shwasanka Jwara*) is usually caused by fever originated Vata imbalances causing inflammation in the lungs (*Vata* organ).

Herbal therapy

Ayurvedic treatment for pneumonia may include herbs like *Uma* or Flaxseeds (V-PK+) and *Nirgundi* or Vitex negundo (VK-P+).

Marmapuncture

Sira	Indication
UB 13	Lung rear organ point. It is used in the treatment of Lung syndromes, especially with fever. Balances the lung.
LI 11	Sea *Sira* (Earth), child of fire, removes the heat especially in LI.
P 6	Bridge point, decreases feelings of hot flushes in the chest.
3D 6	River Point, used in disorders of the thorax (*Kapha* area).

Fever / Headache
GB 20, LI 4, K 7, H 9

Cough / Chest Pain
L 5, L 9

19. Tonsillitis

Tonsillitis (*Tundikeri*) or inflammation of the tonsils is usually caused by the alteration of *Pitta*, affecting the respiratory system.

Herbal therapy

Ayurvedic treatment for tonsillitis may include an herb like *Shatapatri* or Rose flowers (VPK=).

Marmapuncture

Sira	Indication
L 10	Base *Sira*, decreases Fire in Lung.
K 3	Stream *Sira* (Earth). Reduces Fire or heat by acting as its child (of Earth). The Kidney channel runs through the neck/throat, and therefore affects it.
LI 4	Base point of the large intestine (*Vata*). Indicated in discomfort in the area of the throat, by balancing the LI and Lung channels (*Vata*).
LI 11	Sea *Sira* (Earth), child of Fire, removes the heat especially in the LI. Suitable for pharyngeal discomfort, inflammation in the lungs and in the respiratory system.

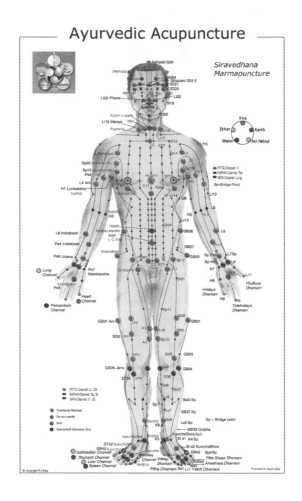

Fig.21. Front chart of the Ayurvedic acupuncture system

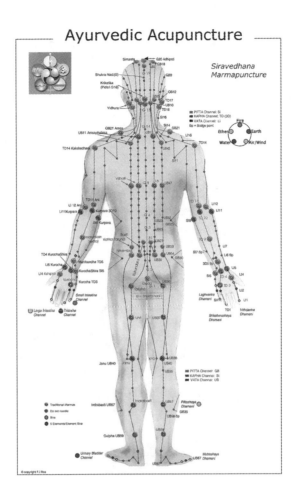

Fig.21B. *Rear chart of the Ayurvedic acupuncture system*
(These charts are available in color full sized from publisher)

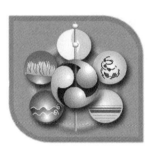

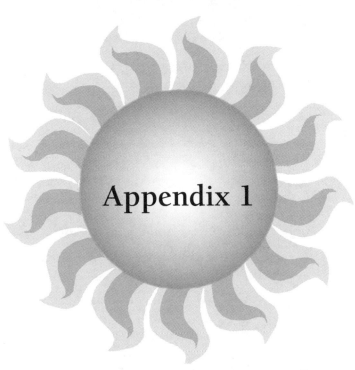

Appendix 1

Marmapuncture siras and their therapeutic effects

Dhamanis of VATA (*PRIMARY*) - Arm

LUNG CHANNEL (Figures 22 and 30)

Channel Name: Phuphusa dhamani
  Organ: Lung *Phuphusa*
  Element: Air / Wind *Vayu*
  Dosha: Vata (Primary)
  Peak Hours Energy: 4 am (between 3-5 am)
  Channel location: Internal part of both arms
  Number of Siras: 11
  Energy Flow: Descending (Ashaya dhamani) *centrifugal*. Transmits Prana to the next Vata channel, the Large Intestine which itself has an ascending flow. The Lung channel (Vata) receives Prana from the previous Pitta dosha channel, the Liver channel which has an ascending flow.
Siras of the Lung Channel- Phuphusa Dhamani Indications and location of the points of Phuphusa dhamani (L): * *asterisk demonstrates siras used often.*

* L 11 (Well, *Kupa* sira, Ether element point, Sira related to Vata with the Well (Air) sira of the Large Intestine channel)
  Location: The point is located at a distance of 0.1 anguli from the radial angle of the nail in the radial border of the thumb.
  Indications: Mental diseases of Vata type as anxiety, nervousness and crying, loss of consciousness, cough, sore throat, nosebleeds, asthma, and febrile illnesses.
  Puncture: The needle is inserted obliquely and shallow upwards to 0.1 anguli depth.

L 10 (Spring, *Sara* sira, Fire element point, sira related to Pitta with the Spring (Water) sira of the Large Intestine channel)
  Location: The point is located in the middle of the first metacarpal on the radial border of it.
  Indications: Fever (Pitta), cough, asthma, hemoptysis, sore and swollen throat.
  Puncture: The needle is inserted perpendicularly to 0.7 anguli depth. Can be treated with *agnikarma*.

* L 9 (Stream, *Sarit* sira and *Mula*-Base point, Earth element point, toni-fication point.) Location: The point is located in the depression in the radial side of the radial artery, next to the trapezius bone and wrist crease.
Indications: Palpitations, cough, sore and swollen throat, asthma, hemoptysis, chest pain, chest tightness, shoulder-arm pain, and inner forearm, dyspnoea.
Puncture: The needle is inserted perpendicularly to 0.7 anguli depth. Can be treated with *agnikarma*.

L 8 (River, *Dhuni* sira, Air / Wind element point related to Vata. Sira which controls PranaVayu)
  Location: The point is located in the depression in the radial side of the radial artery at a distance of 1 anguli above the wrist crease.
  Indications: Cough, sore and swollen throat, sore chest and wrist, asthma.
  Puncture: The needle is inserted perpendicularly to ½ anguli depth.

* L 7 (*Setu*-Bridge point between the Lung and Large Intestine channels. Sira that controls Bhrajaka Pitta)
  Location: The point is located at a distance of 1 ½ anguli in a depression above the wrist crease, at the origin of the radial styloid process.
  Indications: Cough, headache and sore throat, neck stiffness, trismus, weak wrist, facial palsy and asthma.
  Puncture: The needle is inserted obliquely to ½ anguli depth. Can be treated with *agnikarma*.

* L 6 (Cleft, *Antara* sira. Sira that controls Udana Vayu) Part of Indrabasti marma (with TD 9, Sp 4)

Location: The point is located in the antero-inner side of the forearm, 7 angulis above the transverse crease of the wrist, in the line between L 9 and L 5.

Indications: Cough, asthma, pain and inflammation of the throat, pain and loss of function of elbow and arm, tonsillitis, hemoptysis.

Indrabasti Marma Therapy: Stimulates *Agni*, the digestive 'Fire' in the intestinal tract.

Puncture: The needle is inserted perpendicularly to 0.7 anguli depth. Can be treated with *agnikarma*.

* L 5 (Sea, *Samudra* sira, Water element point, sedation point. Sira related to Kapha along with the sira Sea (Earth) of the Large Intestine channel. Sira that controls Bodhaka Kapha and Avalambaka Kapha).

Location: The point is located in the transverse crease of the elbow towards the radial side brachial biceps muscle.

Indications: Cough, asthma, colds, sore and swollen throat, tonsillitis, hemoptysis, vomiting, erysipelas, diarrhea, pain and motor disorders of the elbow and arm.

Puncture: The needle is inserted perpendicularly to ½ anguli depth.

* L 4 Part of Ani marma (together with LI 12 and TD 11)

Location: The point is located in the inner arm, 4 angulis below the tip of the axillary fossa and 1 anguli below L 3.

Indications: Pain in the inside of the arm, sensation of fullness and tightness in the chest, cough.

Ani Marma Therapy: Controls muscle tone.

Puncture: The needle is inserted perpendicularly to ½ anguli depth. Can be treated with *agnikarma*.

L 3 Location: The point is located in the inner arm, 3 angulis below the axillary fold, 6 angulis above L 5.

Indications: Pain in the inner arm, asthma, epistaxis.

Puncture: The needle is inserted perpendicularly to ½ anguli depth.

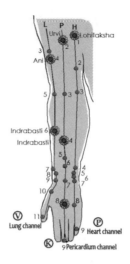

Fig. 22. *Inside arm channels*

L 2

Location: The point is located in the depression, 6 angulis from the midline, or 2 angulis laterally middle of the clavicle.

Indications: Pain and tightness of chest, shoulder and arm pain, back pain, dyspnoea, cough.

Puncture: The needle is inserted perpendicularly to 1 anguli depth. Can be treated with *agnikarma*.

* L 1 (Front point of the Lung and Mamsavaha Srotas)
Apalapa marma

Location: The point is located at a distance of 1 anguli below L 2, 6 angulis from the midline, or 2 angulis laterally middle of the clavicle, at the height of the first intercostal space.

Features: Part of Apalapa marma, making it useful in regulating the autonomic nervous system, "controls Majjavahasrotas (channels of the nervous system)." (Ranade *et al*, *Secrets of Marma*. p. 67)

Indications: Pain and painful oppression of the chest, shoulder and arm pain, dyspnoea, cough.

Apalapa Marma Therapy: Balances the sympathetic and parasympathetic nervous systems.

Puncture: The needle is inserted perpendicularly with the tip pointing outward to ½ anguli depth. Care must be taken when needling the point. Can be treated with *agnikarma*.

LARGE INTESTINE CHANNEL (Figures 23, 26 & 27)

Vata - Arm

Channel Name: Vrihdantra Dhamani
  Organ: Large Intestine *Vrihdantra*
  Element: Air / Wind
  Dosha: Vata (Primary)
  Peak Hours Pranic Energy: 6 am (5-7 am)
  Channel location: Exterior of both arms
  Number of Siras: 20
  Energy Flow: Ascending (Dhatu dhamani) *centripetal*. Receives Prana from the previous Vata channel, Lung, which itself has a descending flow. (From the LI, Prana connects to the next dosha (Kapha) and its Stomach channel).
  Siras of the Vrihdantra dhamani- Large Intestine Indications and location of the points of Vrihdantra dhamani (LI): * *Demonstrates siras used often.*

LI 1 (Well, *Kupa* sira, Wind (Vayu) element point, point related to Vata)
  Location: The point is located in the index finger next to radial side, and 0.1 anguli posteriorly to the nail corner.
  Indications: Loss of consciousness, febrile disease, pain of throat and teeth, swelling in the submandibular area, numbness in the fingers.
  Puncture: The needle is inserted obliquely to 0.1 anguli depth.

LI 2 (Spring, *Sara* sira, Water element point, sedation point. Related to Pitta)
  Location: The point is located in the index finger to the radial side of the second metacarpophalangeal joint of the second metacarpal.
  Indications: Epistaxis, blurred vision, pharyngitis, sore throat and teeth, febrile diseases, lumbago.
  Puncture: The needle is inserted perpendicularly to 0.3 anguli depth. Can be treated with *agnikarma*.

LI 3 (Stream, *Sarit* sira , Ether element point)
  Location: The point is located in the radial side of index finger, in a depression near the head of the second metacarpal bone.
  Indications: Ophthalmic pain, dental and throat pain, swelling and redness of fingers and back of the hand.
  Puncture: The needle is inserted perpendicularly to 1 anguli depth. Can be treated with *agnikarma*.

* LI 4 (*Mula*, Base point of the LI, analgesic point. Sira which controls Ojas)

Kshipra marma

Location: The point is located near the junction of the base of the thumb and forefinger, in the webbing.

Indications: Redness, swelling and ophthalmic pain, headache, sore throat, toothache, epistaxis, motor impairment of the trigeminal nerve, facial paralysis. Febrile disease, sweating, amenorrhea, abdominal pain, constipation, diarrhea, delayed labor.

Kshipra Marma Therapy: Pain of eyes, toothache, redness and pain in the fingers.

Puncture: The needle is inserted perpendicularly to 0.7 anguli depth. Can be treated with *agnikarma*.

LI 5 (River, *Dhuni* sira, Fire element point related to Pitta) Part of Kurccha marma (with TD 3)

Location: The point is located in the depression, radial side of the back of the wrist.

Indications: Pain and swelling of eyes, throat and wrist, headache, toothache.

Kurccha Marma Therapy: Treatment of the large intestine, pain.

Puncture: The needle is inserted perpendicularly to ½ anguli depth. Can be treated with *agnikarma*.

LI 6 (Bridge, *Setu* sira. Bridge point between Large Intestine and Lung channels)

Location: The point is located at a distance of 3 angulis above LI 5, in the line joining LI 5 with LI11, on the outer side of the radius.

Indications: Pain of shoulder, elbow, wrist and arm, edema, epistaxis, deafness.

Puncture: The needle is inserted perpendicularly to ½ anguli depth. Can be treated with *agnikarma*.

LI 7 (Cleft, *Antara* sira)

Location: The point is located at a distance of 2 angulis above LI 6, in the line joining LI 5 with LI 11, on the outer side of the radius.

Indications: Pain of shoulder and arm. Pain and sore throat, headache, abdominal pain, borborygmus, facial edema.

Puncture: The needle is inserted perpendicularly to 0.8 anguli depth. Can be treated with *agnikarma*.

LI 8

Location: The point is located at a distance of 4 angulis below LI 11, on the outer side of the radius.

Indications: Abdominal pain, sore elbow and arm.

Puncture: The needle is inserted perpendicularly to 0.7 anguli depth. Can be treated with *agnikarma*.

LI 9

Location: The point is located at a distance of 3 angulis below LI 11, on the inner side of the radius.

Indications: Paresthesia in hand and arm, pain of shoulder and arm, abdominal pain, bowel sounds, motor impairment in upper limb and head.

Puncture: The needle is inserted perpendicularly to 1 anguli depth. Can be treated with *agnikarma*.

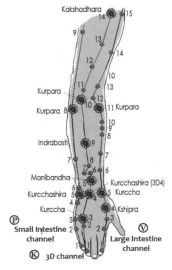

Fig. 23. Outside arm channels

* LI 10

Location: The point is located at a distance of 2 angulis below LI 11, in the line connecting LI 5 with LI 11, on the inner side of the radius.

Indications: Upper limb motor disorders and headaches, vomiting, diarrhea, abdominal pain, shoulder pain.

Puncture: The needle is inserted perpendicularly to 1.2 anguli depth. Can be treated with *agnikarma*.

* LI 11 (Sea, *Samudra* sira, Earth element point, tonification point. Sira related to Kapha along with the Sea (Water) sira of the Lung channel. Sira which controls Ojas)

Part of Kurpara marma (with SI 8 and TD 10)

Location: The point is located in the elbow when flexed at the end of the elbow crease of the inner side of the radius.

Indications: Upper limb motor disorders and headache, sore throat, tonsillitis, fever (cold attack), urticaria, eczema, dermatitis, pruritus, goiter, vomiting, diarrhea, dysentery, scrofula, sore shoulder, arm and elbow, hypertension.

Kurpara Marma therapy: Along with SI 8 and 3D 10 forms part of Kurpara marma and is used in numbness of the arm, elbow pain, cardiac pain, cough, asthma.

Puncture: The needle is inserted perpendicularly to 1 ½ anguli depth. Can be treated with *agnikarma*.

LI 12

Part of Ani marma (with L 4 and TD 11)

Location: The point is located at a distance of an anguli superior to LI 11, on the inner edge of the humerus.

Indications: Numbness, pain and contraction of the elbow and arm.

Ani Marma Therapy: Controls muscle tone.

Puncture: The needle is inserted perpendicularly to anguli ½ depth. Can be treated with *agnikarma*.

LI 13

Location: The point is located 3 angulis above LI 11.

Indications: Scrofula, contraction and pain of elbow and arm.

Puncture: The needle is inserted perpendicularly to 1 anguli depth. Can be treated with *agnikarma*.

* LI 14 Sira which controls Ambhuvaha Srotas.

Location: The point is located at the site where the inferior anterior deltoid muscle end crosses the humerus from the radial side, the line connecting LI 15 with LI 11.

Indications: Upper limb motor disorders and headaches, shoulder and arm, scrofula, lumbago, eye diseases.

Puncture: The needle is inserted perpendicularly to 0.7 anguli depth, taking care not to damage humeral vessels that pass through this area. Can be treated with *agnikarma*.

LI 15

Location: The point is located in the top of the shoulder in the depression between the acromion and the humeral prominence, when raising the arm fully abducted.

Indications: Scrofula, measles, disorders in upper limb motor and head, shoulder and arm pain.

Puncture: The needle is inserted obliquely with the head down to 1 ½ anguli depth. Can be treated with *agnikarma*.

LI 16

Location: The point is located in the depression between the acromial end and the scapular spine.

Indications: Pain and motor impairment of the upper limbs, shoulder pain.

Puncture: The needle is inserted perpendicularly to 0.7 anguli depth. Can be treated with *agnikarma*.

LI 17 Part of Matrika Marma

Location: The point is located in the side of the neck, above the midpoint of the supraclavicular fossa St 12, an anguli below LI 18 point, on the trailing edge of the sternocleidomastoid muscle where the sternal portion of the clavicular portion meet.

Indications: Scrofula, throat inflammation and pain, goiter, hoarseness.

Puncture: The needle is inserted perpendicularly to ½ anguli depth. Can be treated with *agnikarma*.

* LI 18 Sira that controls Raktavaha Srotas.
Part of Manya marma

Location: The point is located at the level of the Adam's apple, on the side of the neck, between the sternal portion and the clavicular portion of the tendon of the sternocleidomastoid muscle.

Indications: Scrofula, swelling and sore throat, goiter, hoarseness, sensation of blockage in the throat, hoarseness, cough, asthma.

Manya Marma Therapy: Is part of Manya marma, which together with the two Nila (St9) are the supraclavicular marmas, which relate to the blood and lymph flow to the head. "*Manya controls Rasa and Rakta vaha srotas also Udana Vata and blood flow.*" (Ranade, *et al*, 1999, 77).

Puncture: The needle is inserted perpendicularly to ½ anguli depth. Can be treated with *agnikarma*.

* LI 19
Part of Phana Marma (with LI 20)
Location: The point is located directly under the edge of the nostril, level with the point G 26, 0.5 anguli away.
Features: Part of Phana marma with LI 20. Controls the sense of smell.
Indications: Deviation of the mouth, epistaxis, nasal obstruction.
Phana Marma Therapy: Runny nose, nasal obstruction and bleeding from the nose.
Puncture: The needle is inserted obliquely to 0.3 anguli depth.

* LI 20
Part of Phana Marma (with LI 19)
Location: The point is located in the naso-labial furrow, at the midpoint of the outer edge of the nostrils, or 0.5 anguli outside edge of the nose.
Indications: Deviation of the mouth, and epistaxis, nasal obstruction, acute rhinitis, chronic allergic, rhinorrhea, anosmia, swelling and itching of the face, facial paralysis and nerve pain, redness, pain in the stomach. Part of Phana marma with LI 19. "*Controls the sense of smell, also controls Vata and Bodhaka Kapha*" (Ranade, *et al*, 1999, p.79).
Phana Marma Therapy: Runny nose, nasal obstruction, and bleeding from the nose.
Puncture: The needle is inserted obliquely to 0.3 anguli depth.

Dhamanis of PITTA (*PRIMARY*) - Arm
HEART CHANNEL (Figures 22 and 30)

Channel Name: Hridaya Dhamani
  Organ: Heart *Hridaya*
  Element: Fire *Tejas*
  Dosha: Pitta (Primary)
  Peak Hours Energy: 12 noon (between 11 am-1 pm)
  Channel location: Interior of both arms
  Number of Siras: 9
  Energy Flow: Descending (Ashaya dhamani) *centrifugal*. Transmits Prana to the next Pitta channel, the Small Intestine, itself having an ascending flow. Heart receives the flow of Prana from the previous Kapha dosha-Spleen channel.

Siras of Hridaya Dhamani-Heart
Indications and location of the points of Hridaya dhamani (C):
* Demonstrates siras used often.

* H 9 (Well, *Kupa* sira, Ether *Akasha* element point, tonification point. Sira related to Vata, together with the Well (Air) sira of the Small Intestine channel)

Location: The point is located in the little finger, radial side, 1 anguli rear of the nail corner.

Indications: Loss of consciousness, mental disorders, chest pain and in the hypochondrium region, palpitation, febrile illnesses.

Puncture: The needle is inserted obliquely to 0.1 anguli depth. Can be treated with *agnikarma*.

* H 8 (Spring, *Sara* sira, Fire *Tejas* element point, Sira related to Pitta with the Spring (Water) sira of the Small Intestine channel)

Location: The point is located between the fourth and fifth metacarpals in the crease on the tip of the little finger when the hand closes.

Indications: Pressure of chest and anxiety, sadness, fear of people, palpitation, shortness of breath, chest pain, enuresis, dysuria, pruritus and pain in the genitals, pain and contracture of the little finger, pain and needle sensation in hands, warmth in the palms, dermal itching.

Puncture: The needle is inserted perpendicularly to 0.3 - ½ anguli depth. Can be treated with *agnikarma*.

* H 7 (Stream, *Sarit* sira, and Base-*Mula* sira, Earth *Prithvi* element point, sedation point. Sira related to Kapha)

Location: The point is located in the rear edge of the pisiform on the wrist crease.

Indications: Hysteria, insomnia, forgetfulness, irritability, mental disorders, epilepsy, chest pain, headache, dizziness, palpitation, irregular menstruation, metrorrhagia, anemia, hemoptysis, dry throat, loss of appetite, feeling of heat in the palms, sores, dermatitis, sudden blindness, yellow sclera, pain in the hypochondrium region.

Puncture: The needle is inserted perpendicularly to 0.3 - ½ anguli depth. Can be treated with *agnikarma*.

* H 6 (Cleft, *Antara* sira)

Location: The point is located at a distance of ½ anguli above the wrist crease on the radial side of the tendon of m. flexor carpi ulnaris.

Indications: Night sweats, hysteria, chest pain.

Puncture: The needle is inserted perpendicularly to 0.3 - ½ anguli depth. Can be treated with *agnikarma*.

* H 5 (Bridge, *Setu* sira. Bridge point between Heart and Small Intestine channels)

Location: The point is located in the antero-inner forearm, 1 anguli above the wrist crease on the radial side of the tendon of flexor carpi ulnaris.

Indications: Aphasia with stiff tongue, hysteria, palpitation, dizziness, vertigo, anxiety, calm or agitated dementia, loss of consciousness, night sweats, sore and swollen throat, sudden hoarseness, enuresis, hematuria, pain in the TM joint, pain in the wrist and arm.

Puncture: The needle is inserted perpendicularly to 0.3 - ½ anguli depth. Can be treated with *agnikarma*.

H 4 (River, *Dhuni* sira, Air/Wind *Vayu* element sira)

Location: The point is located at a distance of 1 ½ anguli above the transverse crease of the wrist on the side of the palm on the radial side of the tendon.

Indications: Contraction of elbow and arm, convulsion, chest pain, sudden hoarseness.

Puncture: The needle is inserted perpendicularly to 0.3 - ½ anguli depth. Can be treated with *agnikarma*.

* H 3 (Sea, *Samudra* sira, Water *Jala* element point. Point related to Kapha along with the Sea (Earth) sira of the Small Intestine channel)

Location: The point is located in the depression between the medial epicondyle of the humerus and the end of transverse crease on the inside of the elbow joint.

Indications: Pain in the axillary region elbow and upper quadrant, chest pain, amnesia, insomnia, calm or agitated dementia, epilepsy, cervical lymphadenopathy, numbness of hands and strong arm tingling sensation, tremor of hand, contraction of the elbow .

Puncture: The needle is inserted perpendicularly to 0.3 - ½ anguli depth. Can be treated with *agnikarma*.

H 2

Location: The point is located 3 angulis above H 3 with the elbow flexed.

Indications: Pain in the hypochondrium region pain, shoulder and arm, yellow sclera.

Puncture: The needle is inserted perpendicularly to 0.3 - ½ anguli depth. Can be treated with *agnikarma*.

H 1

Part of Lohitaksha Marma in the upper limb

Location: The point is located in the center of the axillary region, on the inner side of the axillary artery.

Indications: Scrofula, side and chest pain, cold and painful sensation in the elbow and arm. It is indicated in "hemoptysis, hemiplegia and paraplegia." (Joshi *et al*, 2005, 86)

Therapy of Lohitaksha Marma: Assists circulation and pain in the extremities.

Puncture: The needle is inserted perpendicularly to 0.5-1.0 anguli depth, avoiding the artery. Can be treated with *agnikarma*.

SMALL INTESTINE CHANNEL
(Figures 22, 26 & 27) *Pitta* - Arm

Channel Name: Laghvantra Dhamani

Organ: Small Intestine *Laghvantra*

Element: Fire *Tejas*

Dosha: Pitta (Primary)

Energy Peak Hours: 2 pm (from 1-3pm)

Channel location: Outside of both arms

Number of Siras: 19

Energy Flow: Ascending (Dhatu dhamani) *centripetal*. Receives Prana from its Pitta related channel- the Heart. The Small Intestine transmits Prana to the next Vata channel, Urinary Bladder which itself has a descending flow.

Siras of Laghvantra Dhamani - Small Intestine

Indications and location of the points of Laghvantra Dhamani (ID): * *Demonstrates siras used often.*

SI 1 (Well, *Kupa* sira, Wind / Air *Vayu* element point, Vata related point)

Location: The point is located in the little finger, 0.1 anguli posterior to nail corner.

Indications: Loss of consciousness. Chills and fever without sweating, headache, corneal clouding, stiff tongue, tinnitus, hearing loss, hypogalactia, stiffness and contracture of the neck, lactation deficiency, sore and swollen throat.

Puncture: The needle is inserted obliquely to 0.1 anguli depth. Can be treated with *agnikarma*.

SI 2 (Spring, *Sara* sira, Water *Jala* element point, point related to Pitta. Pitta = Fire and Water)
  Location: The point is located in the front of the fifth metacarpophalangeal articulation, by the back of the hand.
  Indications: Febrile disease, numbness of the fingers.
  Puncture: The needle is inserted perpendicularly to 0.2 - 0.3 anguli depth. Can be treated with *agnikarma*.

* SI 3 (Stream, *Sarit* sira, Ether *Akasha* element point, tonification point. Sira related to Vata)
  Location: The point is located in a depression in the vicinity of the fifth metacarpal head, behind the fifth metacarpophalangeal joint, on the back of the hand.
  Indications: Epilepsy, malaria, night sweats, aphasia after stroke, occipital headache, febrile diseases without sweating, sore and stiff neck, runny eyes, deafness, tinnitus, red and cloudy eyes, twitch contraction of the elbow, arm and fingers, chills.
  Puncture: The needle is inserted perpendicularly to 0.5 -0.7 anguli depth. Can be treated with *agnikarma*.

SI 4 (Base, *Mula* sira)
  Location: The point is located in the depression between the base of the fifth metacarpal bone and triangular (carpometacarpal joint) on the back of the hand.
  Indications: Fever, headache, neck stiffness, clouding of the cornea, pain in the region of hypochondrium.
  Puncture: The needle is inserted perpendicularly to 0.3 - ½ anguli depth. Can be treated with *agnikarma*.

* SI 5 (River, *Dhuni* sira, Fire *Tejas* element point. Sira which controls Samana Vayu and Pachaka Pitta)
Part of Kurccha Shira Marma (with TD 4)
  Location: The point is located in the depression between the ulnar styloid and triangular bone, on the ulnar side of the wrist.
  Indications: Fever, edema of the neck region and sub-mandibular, wrist pain outside the arm. "*Pain and swelling of the dorsum of the hand.*" (Joshi, *et al*, 2005, 48)
  Kurccha Shira Marma Therapy: Heart and lung symptoms.
  Puncture: The needle is inserted perpendicularly to 0.3 - 0.4 anguli depth. Can be treated with *agnikarma*.

* SI 6 (Cleft, *Antara* sira)

 Location: The point is located in the depression between the radial and ulnar extensor carpi ulnaris tendon on the dorsal side of the head of the ulna.

 Indications: Blurred vision, shoulder pain and arm pain, elbow (ulnar) with redness and swelling and inability to raise or lower the hand, low back pain.

 Puncture: The needle is inserted perpendicularly to 0.3 - ½ anguli depth. Can be treated with *agnikarma*.

SI 7 (Bridge, *Setu* sira. Bridge point between Small Intestine and Heart channels). Sira of Jathara Agni.

 Location: The point is located at a distance of 5 angulis above the wrist, the line joining SI 5 and SI 8, in the ulnar border of the ulnar.

 Indications: Mental disorders (panic, fear, sadness, worry), chills and fever, febrile illnesses, neck stiffness, contraction and twitch of the elbow, pain in the fingers, and warts.

 Puncture: The needle is inserted perpendicularly to 0.3 - ½ anguli depth. Can be treated with *agnikarma*.

* SI 8 (Sea, *Samudra* sira, Earth *Prithvi* element point, sedation point. Sira related to Kapha along with the Sea (Water) sira of the Heart Channel) Part of Kurpara Marma (with LI 11 and TD 10)

 Location: The point is located with the elbow flexed, between the olecranon and the medial epicondyle.

 Indications: Epilepsy, pain in the neck and the latero-posterior shoulder, neck and arm, edema on the cheek.

 Kurpara Marma Therapy: Numbness of arm, elbow pain, cardiac pain, cough, asthma.

 Puncture: The needle is inserted perpendicularly to 0.3 – 0.7 anguli depth. Can be treated with *agnikarma*.

* SI 9

 Location: The point is located at a distance of 1 anguli above the end of the posterior axillary fold, with the arm adducted.

 Indications: Motor disorder of the hand and arm, pain in the shoulder region.

 Puncture: The needle is inserted perpendicularly to ½ -1 anguli depth. Can be treated with *agnikarma*.

SI 10

Location: The point is located in the depression inferior-external of the scapular spine, directly above SI 9.

Indications: Pain and weakness of the arm and shoulder.

Puncture: The needle is inserted perpendicularly to 0.8 to 1 anguli depth. Can be treated with *agnikarma*.

SI 11

Location: The point is located in the infrascapular depression, approximately at the level of the fourth thoracic vertebra.

Indications: Pain in the scapula, elbow pain and arm.

Puncture: The needle is inserted obliquely to ½ -1 anguli depth. Can be treated with *agnikarma*.

SI 12

Location: The point is located directly in the depression above SI 11 and the scapula, approximately level with the second thoracic vertebra.

Indications: Pain in the scapular region, numbness and pain in the upper limbs.

Puncture: The needle is inserted perpendicularly to ½ - 0.7 anguli depth. Can be treated with *agnikarma*.

SI 13

Location: The point is located in the internal end of the suprascapular fossa, midway between SI 10 and the spinous process of the second thoracic vertebra.

Indications: Rigidity and pain in the region of the scapula.

Puncture: The needle is inserted obliquely to 0.3 to 0.6 anguli depth. Can be treated with *agnikarma*.

SI 14

Location: The point is located a distance of 3 angulis lateral to the lower edge of the spinous process of the first thoracic vertebra.

Indications: Rigidity of neck, pain of back and shoulder.

Puncture: The needle is inserted obliquely to 0.3 - 0.6 anguli depth. Can be treated with *agnikarma*.

SI 15

Location: The point is located 2 angulis side of the lower border of the spinous process of the seventh cervical vertebra.

Indications: Pain of back and shoulder, cough, asthma.

Puncture: The needle is inserted obliquely from 0.3 - 0.6 anguli depth. Can be treated with *agnikarma*.

SI 16

> **Location**: The point is located on the side of the neck, above and behind LI 18.
>
> **Indications**: Neck rigidity and pain, ringing in the ears, deafness, sore and swollen throat.
>
> **Puncture**: The needle is inserted perpendicularly to ½ -0.8 anguli depth. Can be treated with *agnikarma*.

* SI 17

Part of Matrika Marma (with G 15, TD 16, GB 20 and C 23)

> **Location**: The point is located in the depression behind the angle of the jaw.
>
> **Indications**: Painful and swollen throat, swollen cheek, deafness, ringing noises in the ears.
>
> **Matrika Marma Therapy**: Enhances circulation in the head. Controls Majjavaha Srotas (channels of the nervous system).
>
> **Puncture**: The needle is inserted perpendicularly to ½ -0.8 anguli depth. Can be treated with *agnikarma*.

* SI 18

> **Location**: The point is located in the depression directly below the outer corner of the eye.
>
> **Indications**: Dental pain, tic of the eyelids, yellow sclera, facial paralysis.
>
> **Puncture**: The needle is inserted perpendicularly to ½ -0.8 anguli depth.

* SI 19

> **Location**: The point is located in the depression between the tragus and the jaw joint when the mouth is slightly open.
>
> **Indications**: Panic, tinnitus, deafness, ringing noises in the ears, ear pain and drainage, dental pain, pruritus.
>
> **Puncture**: The needle is inserted perpendicularly to 0.3 - 1 anguli depth. Can be treated with *agnikarma*.

Dhamanis of KAPHA (PRINCIPAL)

STOMACH CHANNEL (Figures 24, 27 and 30) Kapha-Arm

Channel Name: Amashaya Dhamani
  Organ: Stomach *Amashaya*
  Element: Earth *Prithvi*
  Dosha: Kapha (Primary)
  Energy Peak Hours: 8am (between 7-9 am)
  Channel location: In front of both legs, torso and face.
  Number of Siras: 45
  Energy Flow: Descending (Ashaya dhamani) *centrifugal*. Transmits Prana to the next Kapha channel, the Spleen which has an ascending flow. The Stomach channel receives Prana from the previous Vata dosha-Small Intestine channel which itself has an ascending flow.

Siras of the Amashaya dhamani-Stomach

Indications and location of the points of the Amashaya Dhamani (E):
Demonstrates siras used often.

St 45 (Well, *Kupa* sira, Wind / Air *Vayu* element point, sedation point. Sira related to Vata with the Well (Ether) sira of the Spleen Channel)
  Location: The point is located at a distance of 0.1 anguli external side of the second toe.
  Indications: Mental disorders, nightmares, febrile diseases, facial edema, deviation of the mouth, epistaxis, chest tightness and bloating, feeling cold in legs and feet.
  Puncture: The needle is inserted obliquely to 0.1 anguli depth. Can be treated with *agnikarma*.

* St 44 (Spring, *Sara* sira, Water *Jala* element point. Sira related to Pitta with the Spring (Fire) sira of the Spleen channel. Pitta = Fire and Water)
  Location: The point is located in the depression distal and lateral to the second toe.
  Indications: Mental agitation, febrile diseases, toothache, deviation of the mouth, epistaxis, sensation of chest tightness, pain and bloating, diarrhea, dysentery, pain and edema of the dorsum of the foot.
  Puncture: The needle is inserted perpendicularly to 0.3 - ½ anguli *depth. Can be treated with *agnikarma*.

* **St 43 (Stream, *Sarit* sira, Ether *Akasha* element point. Sira related to Vata)**
   Location: The point is located in the depression between the second and third metatarsal bone of the second toe.
   Indications: Edema in the face, dorsum of the foot or general.
   Puncture: The needle is inserted perpendicularly to ½ -0.7 anguli depth. Can be treated with *agnikarma*.

* **St 42 (Base, *Mula* sira)**
Part of the Pada Kurccha Shira Marma (with Sp 5)
   Location: The point is located at a distance of 1.3 angulis distal to St 41, in the depression in the highest part of dorsum of the foot.
   Indications: Inflammation, edema and disorders of the dorsum of the foot. Pada Kurccha Shira Marma therapy: Pain of legs and back, epilepsy.
   Puncture: The needle is inserted perpendicularly to a depth of 0.3 anguli avoiding the artery. Can be treated with *agnikarma*.

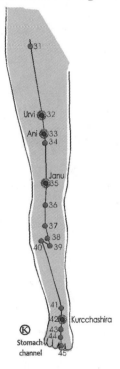

***Fig. 24.** Stomach channel*

* St 41 (River, *Dhuni sira*, Fire *Tejas* element point, tonification point. Sira related to Pitta)

   Location: The point is located on the front of the toe joint in a depression located between the tendon extensor hallucis and the extensor digitorum of the foot.

   Indications: Mental disorders depressive types, pain and paralysis of the lower limbs, headache, dizziness, vertigo.

   Puncture: The needle is inserted perpendicularly to ½ -0.7 anguli depth. Can be treated with *agnikarma*.

* St 40 (Bridge, *Setu sira*. Bridge point between Stomach and Spleen channels)

   Location: The point is located at a distance of 1 anguli externally and lateral to St 38 on the rim of the anterior side of the tibia.

   Indications: Mental disorders and epilepsy, chest pain, cough, asthma, profuse sputum.

   Puncture: The needle is inserted perpendicularly to ½ -1 anguli depth. Can be treated with *agnikarma*.

* St 39

   Location: The point is located at a distance of 3 angulis below St 37.

   Indications: Pain in the lower back, lower abdominal pain, heat in the stomach.

   Puncture: The needle is inserted perpendicularly to ½ -1 anguli depth. Can be treated with *agnikarma*.

* St 38

   Location: The point is located at a distance of 5 angulis below St 36.

   Indications: Pain and paralysis of the legs and shoulder pain.

   Puncture: The needle is inserted perpendicularly to ½ -1 anguli depth. Can be treated with *agnikarma*.

* St 37 (*Sea Point of the Large Intestine in the leg*)

   Location: The point is located at a distance of one anguli out of the front edge of the tibia, 6 angulis below St35.

   Indications: Pain and distended abdomen / large intestine, dysentery, abdominal noises, diarrhea, appendicitis.

   Puncture: The needle is inserted perpendicularly to ½ -1.3 anguli depth. Can be treated with *agnikarma*.

* St 36 (Sea, *Samudra* sira, Earth *Prithvi* element point. Sira related to Kapha along with the Sea (Water) sira of the Spleen channel. Sira which controls Kledaka Kapha and Avalambaka Kapha)

Location: The point is located at a distance of 1 anguli away from the anterior border of the tibia and 3 angulis below St 35.

Indications: Mental disorders, palpitations and nervousness caused by physical weakness (Prana Vayu), sore throat, fever, pain of stomach, vomiting, nausea, abdominal pain, bloating.

Puncture: The needle is inserted perpendicularly to ½ -1.3 anguli depth. Can be treated with *agnikarma*.

* St 35

Part of Janu Marma (with UB 40 and GB 34)

Location: The point is located in the anterolateral aspect of the knee joint in the external depression of the patellar ligament.

Indications: Pain, numbness and motor disturbances of the knee joint.

Janu Marma Therapy: Treats leg and lower back pain, including the hip joint.

Puncture: The needle is inserted obliquely 0.7 to 1 anguli depth, the needle tip is directed slightly toward the inner side. Can be treated with *agnikarma*.

* St 34 (Cleft, *Antara* sira)

Location: The point is located at a distance of 2 angulis above the edge of the kneecap.

Indications: Pain and edema in the knee joint, pain in stomach and bowel.

Puncture: The needle is inserted perpendicularly to ½ -1 anguli depth. Can be treated with *agnikarma*.

St 33

Part of Ani Marma (with GB 31 in addition to -Lv 9 and Sp 10 on the inside of leg)

Location: The point is located at a distance of 3 angulis above the upper outer edge of the patella.

Indications: Pain and motor disorders of the legs, numbness.

Ani Marma Therapy: Controls muscle tone.

Puncture: The needle is inserted perpendicularly to 0.7 -1 anguli depth. Can be treated with *agnikarma*.

* St 32 (Stimulates *Ambhu Vaha Srotas*)
Part of Urvi Marma (with UB 37)
   Location: The point is located in the anterior of the thigh, 6 angulis above
   the upper border of the patella.
   Indications: Paralysis, pain and motor disorders of the legs, cold sensation
   in knees. Pain in the lumbar and iliac regions.
   Urvi Marma Therapy: Stimulates *Ambhu Vaha Srotas*, decreases urinary
   retention and swelling and pain in the groin area.
   Puncture: The needle is inserted perpendicularly to 1 -1 ½ anguli depth.
   Can be treated with *agnikarma*.

* St 31
   Location: The point is located in the depression of the lateral part of the
   sartorius muscle directly below the line of the anterior superior iliac spine
   when the thigh is flexed.
   Indications: Leg numbness and pain, pain or paralysis of the hip and
   thigh, contracture that prevents flexion and extension of the hip, lumbar
   pain and cold in the knees, muscle atrophy.
   Puncture: The needle is inserted perpendicularly to 1 -1 ½ anguli depth.
   Can be treated with *agnikarma*.

St 30
   Location: The point is located at a distance of 2 angulis external to C2
   and 5 angulis below the navel.
   Indications: It harmonizes the stomach, promotes kidney functions, and
   enables Prana.
   Puncture: The needle is inserted perpendicularly to ½ -1 anguli depth.
   Can be treated with *agnikarma*.

* St 29
   Location: The point is located at a distance of 2 angulis external to C3
   and 4 angulis below the navel.
   Indications: Prolapse of the uterus, amenorrhea, leucorrhoea abdominal
   pain, hernia, orchitis.
   Puncture: The needle is inserted perpendicularly to 0.7 - 1.2 anguli depth.
   Can be treated with *agnikarma*.

St 28

Location: The point is located at a distance of 2 angulis external to C4 and 3 angulis below the navel.

Indications: Pain and distension of abdomen (Vata imbalance), hernia, urinary retention, edema, coldness in the bladder, difficult urination, back pain related to menstruation, spine stiffness.

Puncture: The needle is inserted perpendicularly to 0.7 - 1.2 anguli depth. Can be treated with *agnikarma*.

St 27

Location: The point is located at a distance of 2 angulis external to C5 and 2 angulis below the navel.

Indications: Dysuria, hernia, seminal emission, premature ejaculation and lower abdominal distension.

Puncture: The needle is inserted perpendicularly to 0.7 - 1.2 anguli depth. Can be treated with *agnikarma*.

St 26

Location: The point is located at a distance of 2 angulis external to C7 and 1 anguli below the navel.

Indications: Hernia and abdominal pain.

Puncture: The needle is inserted perpendicularly to 0.7 - 1.2 anguli depth. Can be treated with *agnikarma*.

* St 25 (Front point of the Large Intestine and Purishavaha Srotas)

Location: The point is located at a distance of 2 angulis away from the center of the navel.

Indications: Leucorrhea, irregular menstruation, infertility, chronic and acute gastro-enteritis, abdominal pain, noises and bloating in abdomen.

Puncture: The needle is inserted perpendicularly to 0.7 - 1.2 anguli depth. Can be treated with *agnikarma*.

St 24

Location: The point is located at a distance of 2 angulis outside C9 and 1 anguli above the navel.

Indications: Stomach pain, vomiting.

Puncture: The needle is inserted perpendicularly to 0.7 - 1 anguli depth. Can be treated with *agnikarma*.

St 23

Location: The point is located at a distance of 2 angulis from C10 and 2 angulis above the navel.

Indications: Mental disorders like agitation and irritability, indigestion, stomach pain.

Puncture: The needle is inserted perpendicularly to 0.7 - 1 anguli depth. Can be treated with *agnikarma*.

St 22

Location: The point is located at a distance of 2 angulis external to C11 and 3 angulis above the navel.

Indications: Anorexia, edema, abdominal distension and pain signal, noises in the abdomen, diarrhea.

Puncture: The needle is inserted perpendicularly to 0.7 - 1 anguli depth. Can be treated with *agnikarma*.

* St 21

Location: The point is located at a distance of 2 angulis external to C12 and 4 angulis above the navel.

Indications: Anorexia, stomach pain, painful feeling as a "ball" in the epigastrium, vomiting, indigestion, belching, diarrhea.

Puncture: The needle is inserted perpendicularly to 0.7 - 1 anguli depth. Can be treated with *agnikarma*.

St 20

Location: The point is located at a distance of 2 angulis external to C13 and 5 angulis above the navel.

Indications: Anorexia, vomiting, stomach pain, bloating.

Puncture: The needle is inserted perpendicularly to ½ - 1 anguli depth. Can be treated with *agnikarma*.

St 19

Location: The point is located at a distance of 2 angulis lateral to C14 point and 6 angulis above the navel.

Indications: Anorexia, stomach pain, vomiting, abdominal distension.

Puncture: The needle is inserted perpendicularly to ½ -0.7 anguli depth. Can be treated with *agnikarma*.

* St 18

Part of StanaMula marma (with Sp 17, St 17 and K 22)

Location: The point is located one rib below the nipple, in the 5th inter-costal space.

Indications: Cough, dyspnoea, asthma, mastitis, insufficient milk, esoph-ageal stricture with difficulty swallowing, tightness and chest pain, regur-gitation, retching.

Stanamula Marma Therapy: Useful in cough and apnea.

Puncture: The needle is inserted obliquely to 0.3 anguli depth. Can be treated with *agnikarma*.

St 17

Part of Stanamula (with Sp 17, St 18 and K22)

Location: The point is located in the center of the nipple.

Indications: This point is not punctured.

Stanamula Marma Therapy: Useful in cough and apnea.

St 16

Location: The point is located on the mammary line, in the third inter-costal space.

Indications: Mastitis, tightness and chest pain, cough, asthma.

Puncture: The needle is inserted obliquely to 0.3 anguli depth. Can be treated with *agnikarma*.

St 15

Location: The point is located on the mammary line in the second inter-costal space.

Indications: Mastitis, tightness and pain in the chest, cough, asthma.

Puncture: The needle is inserted obliquely to 0.3 anguli depth. Can be treated with *agnikarma*.

St 14

Location: The point is located on the mammary line in the first intercostal space.

Indications: Distension and pain in the hypochondrium region, cough, feeling of oppression and pain in the chest.

Puncture: The needle is inserted obliquely to 0.3 anguli depth. Can be treated with *agnikarma*.

St 13

Location: The point is located on the mammary line in the bottom of the middle of the clavicle.
Indications: Sensation of chest tightness, cough, asthma.
Puncture: The needle is inserted perpendicularly to 0.3 anguli depth. Can be treated with *agnikarma*.

St 12

Location: The point is located at a distance of 4 angulis lateral to Artava Nadi, at the middle point of the supraclavicular fossa.
Indications: Pain in supraclavicular fossa, sore and swollen throat, cough, asthma.
Puncture: The needle is inserted perpendicularly to 0.3 - ½ anguli depth avoiding the artery. It is contraindicated to insert the needle deeply. Can be treated with *agnikarma*.

St 11

Location: The point is located in the upper edge of the inner end of the clavicle.
Indications: Asthma, inflammation and sore throat.
Puncture: The needle is inserted perpendicularly to 0.3 -0.4 anguli depth. Can be treated with *agnikarma*.

St 10

Location: The point is located at a distance of 1 anguli below St9.
Indications: Asthma, inflammation and sore throat.
Puncture: The needle is inserted perpendicularly to 0.3 -0.4 anguli depth. Can be treated with *agnikarma*.

St 9

Part of Nila Marma (with LI 18)

Location: The point is located just next to the carotid artery at the level of the hyoid bone (Adam's apple).
Indications: Asthma, dizziness, flushing and painful inflammation of the throat.
Nila Marma Therapy: Useful in balancing the sense of time and treats hoarseness and loss of taste. "Controls Bhrajaka Pitta, thyroid and brain." (Ranade, *et al*, 1999, p76)
Puncture: The needle is inserted perpendicularly to 0.3 - ½ anguli depth, without puncturing the artery.

* St 8 controls Raktavaha Srotas and Asthivaha Srotas.

Part of Shringataka Marma (with UB 4 and GB 4)

Location: The point is located at a distance of 4 ½ angulis lateral to C 24 and ½ anguli up the front angle at the edge of the hairline.

Indications: Headache caused by cold or heat, vertigo, ophthalmic pain with tearing, tearing caused by the wind, twitching of eyelids, blurred vision.

Shringataka Marma Therapy: Stimulates the nervous system and soothes the eyes, ears, nose and tongue.

Puncture: The needle is inserted horizontally ½ - 1 anguli depth along the scalp with the tip of the needle pointing in a downward direction.

* **St 7**

Location: The point is in the depression directly above St 6, below the edge of the zygomatic arch and anterior to the condyle of the mandible. (The point is located when the patient's mouth is closed).

Indications: Motor disorders of the jaw, temporomandibular joint dislocation, deafness, ringing noises in the ears, otorrhea, facial paralysis, toothache, sore gums, fear of cold wind and not being able to chew.

Puncture: The needle is inserted perpendicularly to 0.3 - ½ anguli depth. Can be treated with *agnikarma*.

* **St 6**

Location: The point is located in the most prominent point of the masseter muscle when teeth are clenched.

Indications: Dental pain, edema of the cheek, facial paralysis, trismus, pain and stiffness of the neck, mumps, fear of cold wind.

Puncture: The needle is inserted perpendicularly to 0.3 - ½ anguli depth or obliquely to the point St 4. Can be treated with *agnikarma*.

* **St 5**

Location: The point is located in the anterior edge of masseter m, 1.3 angulis anterior to the angle of the jaw.

Indications: Dental pain, edema of the cheek, deviation of the mouth, trismus.

Puncture: The needle is inserted obliquely 0.3 anguli depth to the tip of the needle towards the point St 6, do not puncture the artery. Can be treated with *agnikarma*.

* St 4

Location: The point is located at a distance of 0.4 anguli lateral of the mouth.

Indications: Facial paralysis, deviation of the mouth, drooling, tic of the eyelids, facial pain.

Puncture: The needle is inserted obliquely ½ - 1 anguli depth with the tip of the needle to St 6. Can be treated with *agnikarma*.

* St 3

Location: The point is located directly below the pupil and St 2, at the lower edge of the wings of the nose.

Indications: Edema of the lips and cheek, toothache, facial paralysis, tics of the eyelids.

Puncture: The needle is inserted perpendicularly to 0.3 - 0.4 anguli depth. Can be treated with *agnikarma*.

* St 2

Location: The point is located at a distance of less than 0.7 anguli below St 1, in the infraorbital depression.

Indications: Myopia, tic of the eyelids, facial pain, inflammation and eye pain, facial paralysis.

Puncture: The needle is inserted perpendicularly to 0.2 to 0.3 anguli depth. Deep insertion completely contraindicated.

* St 1

Location: The point is located at a distance of 0.7 anguli below the pupil and in the midpoint between the infraorbital rim and the eyeball.

Indications: Myopia, conjunctivitis, eye redness, eyelid twitch, facial paralysis, tearing caused by wind, nystagmus (dancing eyes), night blindness.

Puncture: The needle is inserted perpendicularly to 0.3 - 0.7 anguli depth along the infraorbital edge without rotating the needle.

SPLEEN CHANNEL (Figures 29 and 30)

Kapha - Leg

Channel Name: Pliha Dhamani
  Organ: Spleen *Pliha*
  Element: Earth *Prithvi*
  Dosha: Kapha (Primary)
  Peak Hours Energy: 10am (between 9-11 am)
  Channel location: Interior of both legs
  Number of Siras: 21
  Energy Flow: Ascending (Dhatu dhamani) *centripetal*. Spleen channel receives Prana-from its related dosha -Kapha and the Stomach channel. Transmits Prana to the next Pitta channel, the Heart which itself has a descending flow.

Siras of Pliha Dhamani-Spleen
Indications and location of the points of Pliha Dhamani (Sp):
* *Demonstrates siras used often.*

Sp 1 (Well, *Kupa* sira, Ether *Akasha* element point. Sira related to Vata with the Well (Air) sira of the Stomach channel)
  Location: The point is located at a distance of 0.1 anguli from corner of the nail on the inner side of the big toe.
  Indications: Mental disorders, nightmares, excessive sleepiness, nervousness, sadness, bloating, vomiting, anorexia, diarrhea, epigastric fullness, dyspnoea, chest tightness and heat, uterine bleeding, menorrhagia, hematuria, melaena (intestinal).
  Puncture: The needle is inserted obliquely to 0.1 anguli depth. Can be treated with *agnikarma*.

Sp 2 (Spring, *Sara* sira, Fire *Tejas* element point, tonification point. Sira related to Pitta with the Spring (Water) sira of the Stomach channel)
  Location: The point is located in the inside of the big toe in the anterior part of the first metatarsal phalangeal joint.
  Indications: Nervousness when hungry, febrile diseases without sweating, abdominal distension, vomiting, diarrhea, indigestion, constipation, stomach and back pain, cold extremities, edema in the legs, discomfort caused by moisture.
  Puncture: The needle is inserted perpendicularly to 0.1 -0.2 anguli depth. Can be treated with *agnikarma*.

Sp 3 (Stream, *Sarit* sira, Earth *Prithvi* element point, Base-*Mula* sira. Sira related to Kapha and controls Mamsavaha Srotas).
   Location: The point is located in the inside of the first metatarsal, behind and below the posterior part of the first metatarsophalangeal joint of the big toe.
   Indications: Distension of the chest and hypochondrium, stomach pain, indigestion, bloating, feeling of heaviness in the body (adynamia), dysentery, constipation, vomiting, hemorrhoids, back pain, diarrhea.
   Puncture: The needle is inserted perpendicularly to 0.3 anguli depth. Can be treated with *agnikarma*.

* Sp 4 (Bridge, *Setu* sira. Bridge point between Spleen and Stomach channels)
   Location: The point is located at a distance of 1 anguli from point Sp 3 in the depression in the anteroinferior edge of the first metatarsal.
   Indications: Psychiatric disorders, anxiety, stomach pain, vomiting, borborygmus, abdominal pain, bloating, diarrhea, dysentery, food remains in the feces, menstrual disorders, gynecological disorders.
   Puncture: The needle is inserted perpendicularly to 1 anguli depth. Can be treated with *agnikarma*.

Sp 5 (River, *Dhuni* sira, Wind / Air Vayu element point, sedation point. Sira related to Vata)
Part of Pada Kurccha Shira Marma (with St 42)
   Location: The point is located in depression in the anterior edge of the medial malleolus.
   Indications: Psychiatric disturbances, nervousness, bulimia, headache, stiff and sore tongue, joint pain in foot and ankle, borborygmus, bloating, constipation and abdominal pain, diarrhea, pain in both groin and inner thigh, inguinoscrotal pain radiating to lower abdomen, pain in knees.
   Pada Kurccha Shira Marma Therapy: Pain in legs and back, epilepsy.
   Puncture: The needle is inserted perpendicularly to 0.2 - 0.3 anguli depth. Can be treated with *agnikarma*.

* Sp 6 (Sira which controls Apana Vayu) Apana Sira.
Meeting point (*yoga*) of the channels of Spleen, Liver and Kidney on the leg.
   Location: The point is located at a distance of 3 angulis above the tip of the medial malleolus on the posterior border of the tibia.
   Indications: Insomnia, gastro-intestinal and genito-urinary tract disorders. Pain and paralysis of the legs. Causes Apana vayu to eliminate via the bowel, bladder and uterus.
   Puncture: The needle is inserted perpendicularly to 1 anguli depth. Contraindicated in labor. Can be treated with *agnikarma*.

Sp 7

Location: The point is located at a distance of 3 angulis above Sp 6, 1 finger width from the back edge of the tibia.

Indications: Rigidity of knee and leg paralysis, abdominal distention.

Puncture: The needle is inserted perpendicularly to 0.2 - 1 anguli depth. Can be treated with *agnikarma*.

Sp 8 (Cleft, *Antara* sira)

Location: The point is located in the line joining the point Sp 9 and the medial malleolus, 3 angulis below the medial condyle of the tibia.

Indications: Irregular menstruation and other menstrual disorders (dysmenorrhea, amenorrhea) bloating, hard stomach, hemorrhoids, anorexia, dysentery, dysuria, spermatorrhea, edema, inguinal hernia.

Puncture: The needle is inserted perpendicularly to 1 anguli depth. Can be treated with *agnikarma*.

* Sp 9 (Sea, *Samudra* sira, Water *Jala* element point. Sira related to Kapha along with the Sea (Earth) sira of the Stomach channel)

Location: The point is located in the depression between the posterior border of the tibia and the gastrocnemius muscles.

Indications: Cough, bloating, diarrhea, dysuria, lumbar, knee, leg and foot pain.

Puncture: The needle is inserted perpendicularly to 1 anguli depth. Can be treated with *agnikarma*.

* Sp 10
Part of Ani Marma (with Lv 9, and GB 31 and St 33)

Location: The point is located at a distance of 2 angulis above the superior internal border of the patella.

Indications: Dysmenorrhea, amenorrhea, irregular menstruation, uterine bleeding, knee and inner thigh soreness, urticaria, eczema, erysipelas, psoriasis, herpes zoster, pain, itching and sores on the external genitalia.

Ani Marma Therapy: Controls muscle tone.

Puncture: The needle is inserted perpendicularly to 1 anguli depth. Can be treated with *agnikarma*.

Sp 11

Location: The point is located at a distance of 6 angulis above the point Sp 10.

Indications: Pain and edema in the inguinal region, enuresis and urinary retention.

Puncture: The needle is inserted perpendicularly to ½ anguli depth. Deep insertion is contraindicated. Can be treated with *agnikarma*.

Sp 12

Location: The point is located at a distance of 3 ½ angulis lateral to C2.

Indications: Abdominal pain, cold and fullness, retention of urine, endometriosis, umbilical hernia.

Puncture: The needle is inserted perpendicularly to ½ - 1 anguli depth, taking care since it is located between the nerve and the femoral artery. Can be treated with *agnikarma*.

Sp 13

Location: The point is located at a distance of 4 angulis lateral to the Conception channel and 0.7 anguli above the point Sp 12.

Indications: Inflammation of hypogastrium, abdominal pain, hernia.

Puncture: The needle is inserted perpendicularly to 0.7 - 1 anguli depth. Can be treated with *agnikarma*.

Sp 14

Location: The point is located at a distance of 3 angulis above the point Sp13.

Indications: Diarrhea, pain around the navel.

Puncture: The needle is inserted perpendicularly to ½ - 1 anguli depth. Can be treated with *agnikarma*.

* Sp 15

Location: The point is located directly below the nipple and 4 angulis lateral of the navel.

Indications: Emptiness and coldness in the belly (Vata), dysentery, constipation, indigestion, abdominal pain and coldness.

Puncture: The needle is inserted perpendicularly to ½ - 1 anguli depth. Can be treated with *agnikarma*.

Sp 16

Location: The point is located at a distance of 3 angulis above the point Sp 15.

Indications: Disorders of the abdomen, including constipation, indigestion and dysentery.

Puncture: The needle is inserted perpendicularly to ½ - 1 anguli depth. Can be treated with *agnikarma*.

Sp 17
Part of Stanamula Marma (with St 17, St 18 and K 22)
Location: The point is located in the fifth intercostal space, 2 angulis lateral of the mammary line.

Indications: Pain and pressure in the chest and hypochondrium region. Stanamula Marma Therapy: Useful in cough and apnea.

Puncture: The needle is inserted obliquely 0.3 - ½ anguli depth. Can be treated with *agnikarma*.

Sp 18
Location: The point is located in the fourth intercostal space, 6 angulis lateral to the Conception channel, level with the nipple.

Indications: Deficiency in lactating, cough, pain and tightness in the chest, mastitis.

Puncture: The needle is inserted obliquely 0.4 - ½ anguli depth. Can be treated with *agnikarma* for not more than 10 minutes.

Sp 19
Apastambha Marma
Location: The point is located a rib above the point Sp 18 in the third intercostal space, 6 angulis lateral to the Conception channel.

Indications: Pain and pressure on chest and feeling of fullness and pain in the hypochondrium region, asthma, cough and dyspepsia.

Apastambha Marma Therapy: Asthma, cough and dyspepsia.

Puncture: The needle is inserted obliquely to 0.4 - ½ anguli depth. Can be treated with *agnikarma*.

Sp 20
Stanya Rohita Marma
Location: The point is located in the second intercostal space, 6 angulis lateral to the Conception channel.

Indications: Chest pain and tightness, pain in the hypochondrium region, feeling of fullness.

Stanya Rohita Marma Therapy: Numbness in arms.

Puncture: The needle is inserted obliquely to 0.4 - ½ anguli depth. Can be treated with *agnikarma*.

Sp 21 (Bridge, Setu sira. Bridge point that has effect on all the inner pranic ducts which form bridges or platforms between their related dhamanis)
Location: The point is located halfway between the armpit and the end of the eleventh rib, 6 angulis below the armpit.

Indications: Pain throughout the body and limb weakness (asthenia), pain in the chest and in the hypochondrium region, asthma.

Puncture: The needle is inserted obliquely to 0.3 - ½ anguli depth. Can be treated with *agnikarma*.

Dhamanis of VATA (*SECONDARY*) - Leg

URINARY BLADDER CHANNEL (Figures 25, 26 and 27)

Channel Name: Mutrashaya Dhamani
  Organ: Urinary Bladder   *Mutrashaya*
  Element: Water (-) *Jala*
  Dosha: Vata (Secondary)
  Energy Peak Hours: 2pm (1-3 pm)
  Channel location: Back of body and legs.
  Number of Siras: 67
  Travel: Head, back of the torso, leg.
  Energy Flow: Descending (Ashaya dhamani) *centrifugal*. The Urinary Bladder channel transmits Prana to the next related Vata channel, the Kidney which itself has an ascending flow. The Urinary Bladder channel receives Prana from the previous dosha Pitta- the Small Intestine channel.

Siras of Mutrashaya Dhamani-Urinary Bladder
Indications and location of the points of Mutrashaya dhamani (UB):
* Demonstrates siras used often.

* UB 67 (Well, *Kupa* sira, Wind / Air *Vayu* element point, tonification point. Sira related to Vata with the Well sira (Ether) of the Kidney Channel)
  Location: The point is located in the root of the nail corner 0.5 anguli to outer side of the little toe.
  Indications: Difficult labor and fetal malposition, sore neck and eye, headache, epistaxis, nasal obstruction, sensation of heat on the soles of the feet.
  Puncture: The needle is inserted superficially and obliquely to 0.1 anguli depth. Can be treated with *agnikarma*.

UB 66 (Spring, *Sara* sira, Water *Jala* element point. Sira related to Pitta with the Spring (Fire) sira of the Kidney Channel)
  Location: The point is located in the outer edge of the foot, in a depression below and forward of the metatarsophalangeal joint of the 5th toe.
  Indications: Spasms and fever, blurred vision, headache, epistaxis, nasal obstruction, stiff neck, body aches, sub-lingual swelling that causes speech difficulty.
  Puncture: The needle is inserted perpendicularly to 0.2 anguli depth. Can be treated with *agnikarma*.

UB 65 (Stream, *Sarit* sira, Ether *Akasha* element point, sedation point. Sira related to Vata)

Location: The point is located in a depression between the head and body of the 5th metatarsus, on the outer edge of the dorsum of the foot.

Indications: Headache, blurred vision, mental confusion, nasal obstruction, stiff neck, back and hip pain, boils and sores on the back, pain in the back of the thighs, heat and pain of body, heat in the sole of the foot.

Puncture: The needle is inserted perpendicularly to 0.3 anguli depth. Can be treated with *agnikarma*.

UB 64 (Base, *Mula* sira of the Urinary Bladder)

Location: The point is located below the 5th metatarsal protuberance, and in the outer edge of the foot.

Indications: Headache, stiff neck, blurred vision, epilepsy, vertigo, diarrhea, rashes and sores on the feet, lower back pain and leg pain.

Puncture: The needle is inserted perpendicularly to ½ anguli depth. Can be treated with *agnikarma*.

UB 63 (Cleft, *Antara* sira)

Location: The point is located in the outer depression cuboid, and antero-inferior to UB 62.

Indications: Convulsion child epilepsy, back pain, movement disorders and pain in legs.

Puncture: The needle is inserted perpendicularly to ½ anguli depth. Can be treated with *agnikarma*.

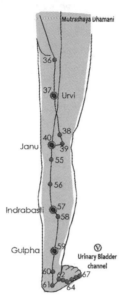

Fig. 25. *Urinary bladder channel*

* UB 62

Location: The point is located at a distance of ½ anguli directly below the lower edge of the lateral malleolus in the depression.
Indications: Mental disturbances, insomnia, dizziness, epilepsy, headache, tinnitus, symptoms of hemiplegia, back pain, leg pain.
Puncture: The needle is inserted perpendicularly to 0.3 anguli depth. Can be treated with *agnikarma*.

UB 61

Location: The point is located in the depression of the calcaneus, at the lower part of the lateral malleolus (directly below UB 60).
Indications: Pain of heel, muscle atrophy and weakness of the legs.
Puncture: The needle is inserted perpendicularly to ½ anguli depth. Can be treated with *agnikarma*.

* UB 60 (River, *Dhuni* sira, Fire *Tejas* element point. Sira related to Pitta).

Location: The point is located midway between the external protuberance of the medial malleolus and the calcaneal tendon, in the depression that exists there.
Indications: Difficult labor, epilepsy in children, headache, blurred vision, stiff neck, sciatica, spasm and shoulder, arm, back, heel and ankle pain.
Puncture: The needle is inserted perpendicularly to ½ anguli depth. *Contraindicated in pregnancy.* Can be treated with *agnikarma*.

* UB 59
Part of Gulpha Marma (with GB39)
   Location: The point is located 3 angulis directly above UB 60.
   Indications: Sensation of light-headedness, headache, kidney and bladder inflammation, lumbago, paralysis of the legs, swelling and edema of the lateral malleolus, rheumatoid arthritis.
   Gulpha Marma Therapy: Treatment of paralysis and pain of the leg (especially in the ankle joint).
   Puncture: The needle is inserted perpendicularly to 1 anguli depth. Can be treated with *agnikarma*.

* UB 58 (Bridge, *Setu* sira. Bridge point between Urinary Bladder and Kidney channels)
   Location: The point is located at a distance of 7 angulis directly above UB60, and in the rear edge of the fibula.
   Indications: Blurred vision, headache, nasal obstruction, leg weakness, lumbago.
   Puncture: The needle is inserted perpendicularly to 1 anguli depth. Can be treated with *agnikarma*.

* UB 57
Part of Indrabasti Marma. Sira of Jathara Agni and Anna Vaha Srotas.
   Location: The point is located directly below the gastrocnemius muscle (in the separation of the inner and outer ends) in the line joining point UB 40 with the calcaneal tendon.
   Indications: Neuropathy, lumbago, rectal prolapse, hemorrhoids, constipation, muscle cramps.
   Indrabasti Marma therapy: Stimulates *Agni*, the digestive 'Fire' in the intestinal tract.
   Puncture: The needle is inserted perpendicularly to 1 anguli depth. Can be treated with *agnikarma*.

UB 56
   Location: The point is located in the center of the gastrocnemius muscle, between the points UB 55 and UB 57.
   Indications: Acute lumbago, leg pain, hemorrhoids.
   Puncture: The needle is inserted perpendicularly to 1 anguli depth. Can be treated with *agnikarma*.

UB 55
   Location: The point is located between the inner and outer ends of the calf muscles, 2 angulis directly below the point UB 40.
   Indications: Lumbago, pain, numbness and paralysis of the legs.
   Puncture: The needle is inserted perpendicularly to 1 anguli depth. Can be treated with *agnikarma*.

* UB 54
Part of Nitamba Marma
  Location: The point is located at a distance of 3 angulis out from Shukra
  Channel, at the sacral foramen level.
  Indications: Sciatica, movement disorders and pain in the legs and lum-
  bosacral region, hemorrhoids, muscle atrophy.
  Nitamba Marma Therapy: Pain in the lower back, sciatica, paralysis of
  lower extremities, bowel problems. Nitamba Marma controls Rasavaha
  and Asthivaha srotas. (Lele, et al, 1999, 71).
  Puncture: The needle is inserted perpendicularly to 1 anguli depth. Can
  be treated with *agnikarma*.

UB 53
Part of Katika Taruna Marma (with UB31)
  Location: The point is located at the level of the lower border of the spinous
  process of the second sacral vertebra, three angulis out.
  Indications: Lumbago, abdominal distention and noises.
  Katika Taruna Marma Therapy: Treatment of the hip joint. Controls
  Asthivaha and Swedavaha srotas. Bhrajaka is related to Pitta.
  Puncture: The needle is inserted perpendicularly to 1 anguli depth. Can
  be treated with *agnikarma*.

UB 52
  Location: The point is located at the level of the lower border of the spinous
  process of the second lumbar vertebra, three angulis out.
  Indications: Rigidity, edema and pain in the lumbar region, seminal emission and impotence, dysuria.
  Puncture: The needle is inserted perpendicularly to 1 anguli depth. Can
  be treated with *agnikarma*.

UB 51
  Location: The point is located at the level of the lower border of the spinous process of the first lumbar vertebra, three angulis out.
  Indications: Pain of neck and legs, pain in the epigastric region, constipation, abdominal tumor.
  Puncture: The needle is inserted perpendicularly to 1 anguli depth. Can
  be treated with *agnikarma*.

UB 50
  Location: The point is located at the level of the lower border of the spinous
  process of the twelfth thoracic vertebra, three angulis out. Indications: Back
  pain, pain in the epigastric region, abdominal distension.
  Puncture: The needle is inserted obliquely to ½ anguli depth. Can be
  treated with *agnikarma*.

UB 49

Location: The point is located at the level of the lower border of the spinous process of the eleventh thoracic vertebra, 3 angulis out.

Indications: Dysphagia, lumbago, sciatica, cystitis, vomiting, bloating and abdominal noises, diarrhea, hemorrhoids.

Puncture: The needle is inserted obliquely to ½ anguli depth. Can be treated with *agnikarma*.

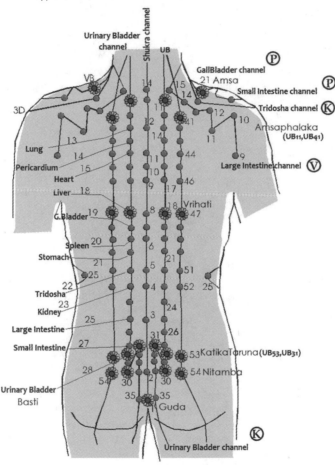

Fig. 26. Rear torso channels

UB 48

Location: The point is located at the level of the lower border of the spinous process of the tenth thoracic vertebra, three angulis out.

Indications: Jaundice, borborygmus, bloating and abdominal pain, diarrhea.

Puncture: The needle is inserted obliquely to ½ anguli depth. Can be treated with *agnikarma*.

UB 47
Part of Vrihati Marma (with UB 18)
   Location: The point is located at the level of the lower border of the spinous process of the ninth thoracic vertebra, three angulis out.
   Indications: Vomiting, diarrhea, back pain, chest and hypochondrium.
   Vrihati Marma Therapy: Coughing up blood, cardiac symptoms.
   Puncture: The needle is inserted obliquely to 1 anguli depth. Can be treated with *agnikarma*.

UB 46
   Location: The point is located at the level of the lower border of the spinous process of the seventh thoracic vertebra, three angulis out.
   Indications: Dysphagia, pain and stiffness in the back, vomiting, belching.
   Puncture: The needle is inserted obliquely to ½ anguli depth. Can be treated with *agnikarma*.

UB 45
   Location: The point is located at the level of the lower border of the spinous process of the sixth thoracic vertebra, 3 angulis out.
   Indications: Pain and / or stiffness of shoulder and back, asthma, cough.
   Puncture: The needle is inserted obliquely to ½ anguli depth. Can be treated with *agnikarma*.

UB 44
   Location: The point is located at the level of the lower border of the spinous process of the fifth thoracic vertebra, 3 angulis out.
   Indications: Pain and / or stiffness of shoulder and back, asthma, cough.
   Puncture: The needle is inserted obliquely to ½ anguli depth. Can be treated with *agnikarma*.

UB 43
   Location: The point is located at the level of the lower border of the spinous process of the fourth thoracic vertebra, 3 angulis out.
   Indications: Amnesia, night sweats, pulmonary tuberculosis, asthma, cough, hemoptysis, indigestion, abnormal seminal emission.
   Puncture: The needle is inserted obliquely to ½ anguli depth. Can be treated with *agnikarma*.

UB 42

Location: The point is located at the level of the lower border of the spinous process of the third thoracic vertebra, 3 angulis out.

Indications: Pain in the shoulder and back, neck stiffness, cough, pulmonary tuberculosis, asthma.

Puncture: The needle is inserted obliquely to ½ anguli depth. Can be treated with *agnikarma*.

* UB 41

Part of Amsaphalaka Marma (with UB 11), Fourth Chakra

Location: The point is located at the level of the lower border of the spinous process of the second thoracic vertebra, 3 angulis out.

Indications: Paresthesia and / or numbness of the elbow and arm, stiffness and pain in shoulder, back and neck.

Amsaphalaka Marma Therapy: Is used to treat shoulder pain and the Fourth Chakra (chest).

Puncture: The needle is inserted obliquely to ½ anguli depth. Can be treated with *agnikarma*.

* UB 40 (Sea, *Samudra* sira, Earth *Prithvi* element point. Point related to Kapha along with the Sea (Water) sira of the Kidney channel), sira which controls Ambhu vaha Srotas.

Part of Janu Marma (with GB 34 and St 35)

Location: The point is located in the midpoint of the popliteal transverse crease.

Indications: Motor impairment and pain in leg and hip, abdominal pain, vomiting, diarrhea, lumbago, contraction of the tendons of the popliteal zone, muscular atrophy, hemiplegia, skin and genito-urinary tract disorders.

Janu Marma Therapy: Treats pain in the legs and lower back, including the hip joint.

Puncture: The needle is inserted perpendicularly to 1 anguli depth.

UB 39

Location: The point is located in the inner edge of the tendon of the biceps femoris, outside UB 40.

Indications: Distention of the lower abdomen (Vata area), dysuria, pain and stiffness in the lower back, leg and foot.

Puncture: The needle is inserted perpendicularly to 1 anguli depth. Can be treated with *agnikarma*.

UB 38
Location: The point is located in the inside of the biceps femoris tendon at a distance of one anguli above UB 39.
Indications: Paresthesia in the thigh, contraction of the tendons in the popliteal area, numbness in the femoral and gluteal areas.
Puncture: The needle is inserted perpendicularly to 1 anguli depth. Can be treated with *agnikarma*.

* UB 37

Part of Urvi marma (with St 32)
Location: The point is located in the center of the back of the thigh, the line connecting the points UB 36 and UB 40.
Indications: Lumbago and thigh pain, urine retention.
Urvi marma therapy: Stimulates *Ambhu Vaha Srotas*, so it is used in urinary retention and edema and pain in the groin area.
Puncture: The needle is inserted perpendicularly to 1 anguli depth. Can be treated with *agnikarma*.

* UB 36 (Sira which controls Mutravaha Srotas)
Location: The point is located in the middle of the gluteal fold.
Indications: Pain in the lumbar, sacral, gluteal areas and femoral arteries, hemorrhoids.
Puncture: The needle is inserted perpendicularly to 1 anguli depth. Can be treated with *agnikarma*.

UB 35 (Local sira controlling Apana Vayu)
Location: The point is located at a distance of ½ anguli out from the Shukra Channel lateral to the tip of the coccyx.
Indications: Hemorrhoids, diarrhea, dysentery, leucorrhea, impotence.
Puncture: The needle is inserted perpendicularly to 1 anguli depth. Can be treated with *agnikarma*.

UB 34
Location: The point is located between the point UB 30 and the Shukra channel, at the level of the fourth foramen of the sacrum.
Indications: Lumbago, lower abdominal pain (hypogastrium), constipation, dysuria and urinary retention.
Puncture: The needle is inserted perpendicularly to 1 anguli depth. Can be treated with *agnikarma*.

UB 33

Location: The point is located between the point UB 29 and the Shukra channel, at the level of the third foramen of the sacrum.

Indications: Sciatica, lumbago, constipation, dysuria, irregular menstruation, leucorrhea, hemorrhoids.

Puncture: The needle is inserted perpendicularly to 1 anguli depth. Can be treated with *agnikarma*.

* UB 32 (Local sira controlling Apana Vayu)

Location: The point is located in the midpoint between the top edge of the iliac spine and the Shukra channel, at the level of the second foramen of the sacrum.

Indications: Local point of Apana vayu. Lumbago, sciatica, rheumatism, muscular atrophy, motor disorders of the legs, hernia, irregular menstruation, leucorrhea, hemorrhoids.

Puncture: The needle is inserted perpendicularly to 1 anguli depth. Can be treated with *agnikarma*.

UB 31

Part of Katika Taruna Marma (with UB 53)

Location: The point is located in the midpoint between the top edge of the iliac spine and the Shukra channel, at the level of the first foramen of the sacrum.

Indications: Lumbago, sciatica, prolapsed uterus, irregular menstruation, leucorrhea, constipation, hemorrhoids, scanty urine.

Katika Taruna Marma Therapy: Treatment of the hip joint.

Puncture: The needle is inserted perpendicularly to 1 anguli depth. Can be treated with *agnikarma*.

UB 30 (Sira which controls Mutravaha Srotas)

Location: The point is located at a distance of 1 ½ anguli out from the Shukra channel, at the level of the fourth foramen of the sacrum.

Indications: Lumbago, pain in the hip joints, abnormal seminal emission, irregular menstruation, leucorrhea, endometriosis, hernia.

Puncture: The needle is inserted perpendicularly to 1 anguli depth.

UB 29

Location: The point is located at a distance of 1 ½ angulis outward from the Shukra channel, at the level of the third foramen of the sacrum.

Indications: Pain and stiffness in the lumbar region, dysentery, hernia.

Puncture: The needle is inserted perpendicularly to 1 anguli depth. Can be treated with *agnikarma*.

* UB 28 (Rear point of the Urinary Bladder and Mutravaha Srotas)
Part of Basti marma (with C. 4 and C 6)
   Location: The point is located at a distance of 1 ½ anguli outward from the Shukra channel, at the level of the second foramen of the sacrum.
   Indications: Pain and stiffness in the lumbar region, retention of urine, spermatorrhea, and enuresis, diarrhea, constipation, abdominal pain and bloating.
   Basti Marma Therapy: Diseases of the genitourinary tract.
   Puncture: The needle is inserted perpendicularly to 1 anguli depth. Can be treated with *agnikarma*.

* UB 27 (Rear point of the Small Intestine and Artavavaha Srotas)
   Location: The point is located at a distance of 1 ½ angulis outward from the Shukra channel, at the level of the first foramen of the sacrum.
   Indications: Pain and lower abdominal distension, enuresis, dysentery, abnormal seminal emission, hematuria.
   Puncture: The needle is inserted perpendicularly to 1 anguli depth. Can be treated with *agnikarma*.

UB 26
   Location: The point is located at a distance of 1 ½ anguli out from the Shukra channel, below the spinous process of the fifth lumbar vertebra.
   Indications: Lumbago, diarrhea, abdominal distension.
   Puncture: The needle is inserted perpendicularly to 1 anguli depth. Can be treated with *agnikarma*.

* UB 25 (Rear point of the Large Intestine and Purishavaha Srotas)
   Location: The point is located at a distance of 1 ½ anguli out from the bottom edge of the spinous process of the fourth lumbar vertebra.
   Indications: Paralysis in children, lumbago, pain and bloating, enteritis, diarrhea, constipation.
   Puncture: The needle is inserted perpendicularly to 1 anguli depth. Can be treated with *agnikarma*.

UB 24
   Location: The point is located at a distance of 1 ½ anguli out from the bottom edge of the spinous process of the third lumbar vertebra.
   Indications: Lumbago, back pain, hemorrhoids.
   Puncture: The needle is inserted perpendicularly to 1 anguli depth. Can be treated with *agnikarma*.

* **UB 23 (Rear point of the Kidney and Medovaha Srotas)**
Location: The point is located at a distance of 1 ½ anguli out the bottom edge of the spinous process of the second lumbar vertebra.
Indications: Deafness, tinnitus, blurred vision, back pain, abnormal seminal emission, impotence, enuresis, irregular menstruation, leucorrhea, weakness in the knees, edema, pain in the feet. It is very useful in chronic conditions.
Puncture: The needle is inserted perpendicularly to 1 anguli depth. Can be treated with *agnikarma*.

* **UB 22 (Rear point of Tridosha and Shukravaha Srotas)**
Location: The point is located at a distance of 1 ½ anguli out from the bottom edge of the spinous process of the first lumbar vertebra.
Indications: Pain and stiffness of the lumbar region, vomiting, bloating, indigestion, diarrhea, dysentery, edema.
Puncture: The needle is inserted perpendicularly to 1 anguli depth. Can be treated with *agnikarma*.

* **UB 21 (Rear point of the Stomach and Annavaha Srotas)**
Location: The point is located at a distance of 1 ½ anguli out from the bottom edge of the spinous process of the twelfth thoracic vertebra.
Indications: Abdominal distention, nausea, indigestion, pain in chest, epigastric and hypochondrium, vomiting.
Puncture: The needle is inserted obliquely to ½ anguli depth. Can be treated with *agnikarma*.

* **UB 20 (Rear point of the Spleen and Udakavaha Srotas)**
Location: The point is located at a distance of 1 ½ anguli out from the bottom edge of the spinous process of the eleventh thoracic vertebra.
Indications: Anorexia, fatigue, pain and inflammation of the back, vomiting, indigestion, abdominal distension, jaundice, dysentery, diarrhea, weight loss despite eating a lot, sore throat, pain accompanied by cold, edema.
Puncture: The needle is inserted obliquely to ½ anguli depth. Can be treated with *agnikarma*.

* **UB 19 (Rear point of the Gallbladder and Raktavaha Srotas)**
Location: The point is located at a distance of 1 ½ anguli out from the bottom edge of the spinous process of the tenth thoracic vertebra.
Indications: Insomnia, afternoon fever, bitter taste in the mouth (Pitta), pain in the chest and hypochondrium, jaundice, gagging, pulmonary tuberculosis.
Puncture: The needle is inserted obliquely to ½ anguli depth. Can be treated with *agnikarma*.

* UB 18   (Rear point of the Liver and Raktavaha Srotas)
Part of Vrihati Marma (with UB 47)
  Location: The point is located at a distance of 1 ½ anguli out from the bottom edge of the spinous process of the ninth thoracic vertebra.
  Indications: Mental disorders and epilepsy, blurred vision, conjunctivitis, epistaxis, jaundice, pain in the back and hypochondrium, hematemesis, hemeralopia (day blindness).
  Vrihati Marma Therapy: Cough with blood, cardiac symptoms.
  Puncture: The needle is inserted obliquely to ½ anguli depth. Can be treated with *agnikarma*.

* UB 17
  Location: The point is located at a distance of 1 ½ anguli out from the bottom edge of the spinous process of the seventh thoracic vertebra.
  Indications: Swallowing difficulty, evening fever (Vata type), night sweats, vomiting, cough, hiccough, asthma, hemoptysis, leukemia, lethargy, not wanting to talk, widespread pain, dysphagia.
  Puncture: The needle is inserted obliquely to ½ anguli depth. Can be treated with *agnikarma*.

UB 16
  Location: The point is located at a distance of 1 ½ anguli out from the bottom edge of the spinous process of the sixth thoracic vertebra.
  Indications: Chest and abdominal pain.
  Puncture: The needle is inserted obliquely to ½ anguli depth. Can be treated with *agnikarma*.

* UB 15 (Rear point of the Heart and Pranavaha Srotas)
  Location: The point is located at a distance of 1 ½ anguli out from the bottom edge of the spinous process of the fifth thoracic vertebra.
  Indications: Amnesia, palpitation, tachycardia, panic, irritability, chest pain, shocks, hemoptysis, epilepsy, cough.
  Puncture: The needle is inserted obliquely to ½ anguli depth. Can be treated with *agnikarma*.

* UB 14 (Rear point of the Pericardium and Rasavaha Srotas)
  Location: The point is located at a distance of 1 ½ anguli out from the bottom edge of the spinous process of the fourth thoracic vertebra.
  Indications: Mental agitation, heart disease, sensation of tightness in the chest.
  Puncture: The needle is inserted obliquely to ½ anguli depth. Can be treated with *agnikarma*.

* UB 13 (Rear point of the Lung and Mamsavaha Srotas)

Location: The point is located at a distance of 1 ½ anguli out from the bottom edge of the spinous process of the third thoracic vertebra.

Indications: Vata type fever, night sweats, lung disorders, thirst, chest tightness and hypochondrium distension with not wanting to eat, itching of the skin, contraction of the back.

Puncture: The needle is inserted obliquely to ½ anguli depth. Can be treated with *agnikarma*.

UB 12

Location: The point is located at a distance of 1 ½ anguli out from the bottom edge of the spinous process of the second thoracic vertebra.

Indications: Headache, stiff neck, cold, cough, fever, back pain, heat in the chest, skin disorders on the back.

Puncture: The needle is inserted obliquely to ½ anguli depth. Can be treated with *agnikarma*.

* UB 11

Part of Amsaphalaka Marma (with UB 41), Fourth Chakra (*Anahata*)

Location: The point is located at a distance of 1 ½ anguli out from the bottom edge of the spinous process and the first thoracic vertebra.

Indications: Arthritis of the joints, pain in the shoulder, neck stiffness, cough, fever, headache.

Amsaphalaka Marma Therapy: It is used to treat the Fourth Chakra (Anahata).

Puncture: The needle is inserted obliquely to ½ anguli depth. Can be treated with *agnikarma*.

UB 10

Location: The point is located at a distance of ½ anguli the rear edge of the scalp, at a distance of 1.3 anguli outwards from the Shukra channel (G 15).

Indications: Vertigo and dizziness, headache, and stiff neck with fear to the wind, pain in the shoulder and back, decreased visual acuity, lacrimation, anosmia, epilepsy and childhood seizure, nasal obstruction.

Puncture: The needle is inserted perpendicularly to ½ anguli depth. Can be treated with *agnikarma*.

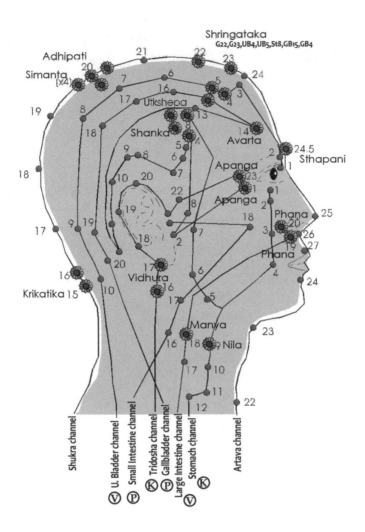

Fig. 27. Head channels

UB 9

Location: The point is located in the outer side of the upper edge of the occiput, at a distance of 1.3 anguli outside the Shukra channel (G 17).
Indications: Headache, eye pain, nasal obstruction.
Puncture: The needle is inserted horizontally to ½ anguli depth.

UB 8

Location: The point is located at a distance of 1 ½ angulis out form the Shukra channel, posterior to the point UB 7.
Indications: Mental disorders, dizziness, tinnitus.
Puncture: The needle is inserted horizontally to ½ anguli depth.

UB 7

Location: The point is located at a distance of 1 ½ anguli out from the Shukra channel, 1 ½ angulis posterior to the point UB6, 4 angulis above the hairline.

Indications: Rhinorrhea, nasal polyps, dizziness, headache, nasal obstruction, epistaxis.

Puncture: The needle is inserted horizontally to ½ anguli depth.

UB 6

Location: The point is located at a distance of 1 ½ anguli outside the Shukra channel, at a distance of 1 ½ anguli posterior to UB 5.

Indications: Obstruction of nose, blurred vision, headache.

Puncture: The needle is inserted horizontally to ½ anguli depth.

* UB 5

Part of the 2nd Shringataka Marma (with GB 15, G 22 and G 23)

Location: The point is located at a distance of one anguli within the hairline, above UB 4.

Indications: Blurred vision, epilepsy, headache.

Shringataka Marma Therapy: Stimulates the nervous system and soothes the eyes, ears, nose and tongue.

Puncture: The needle is inserted horizontally to ½ anguli depth.

* UB 4

Part of 1st Shringataka Marma (with GB 4, St 8)

Location: The point is located at a distance of 1 ½ anguli lateral to point G 24.

Indications: Blurred vision, sore eyes, front and vertex headache, epistaxis, nasal obstruction.

Shringataka Marma Therapy: Stimulates the nervous system and soothes the eyes, ears, nose and tongue.

Puncture: The needle is inserted horizontally to ½ anguli depth.

UB 3

Location: The point is located between points G 24 and UB 4, above the internal end of the eyebrow.

Indications: Epilepsy, dizziness, headache.

Puncture: The needle is inserted horizontally to ½ anguli depth.

* **UB 2**
 Location: The point is located in the depression, medial end of eyebrow.
 Indications: Blurred vision, dizziness, headache, pain in the supra orbital region, tearing caused by wind, conjunctivitis, eyelid tic, myopia.
 Puncture: The needle is inserted horizontally to ½ anguli depth towards UB1 or towards the center of the eyebrow.

* **UB 1**
 Location: The point is located 0.1 anguli from the inner corner of the eye. To locate this point the patient must close the eyes.
 Indications: Disorders of the eyes. Dangerous point.
 Puncture: 6 mm. Superficial only.

KIDNEY CHANNEL (Figures 28, 29 and 30)
Vata-Leg

Channel Name: Vrikka Dhamani
 Organ: Kidney *Vrikka*
 Element: Water (-) *Jala*
 Dosha: Vata (Secondary)
 Energy Peak Hour: 4 pm (between 5-7 pm)
 Channel location: Interior of both legs
 Number of Siras: 27
 Energy Flow: Ascending (Dhatu dhamani) *centripetal*. Prana is transmitted to the next channel-Kapha dosha-the Pericardium channel that itself has an ascending flow. The Kidney channel receives the flow of Prana from its Vata-related -the Urinary Bladder channel which itself has a descending flow.

Siras of the Vrikka Dhamani-Kidney
Indications and location of the points of Vrikka dhamani (K): * *Demonstrates siras used often.*

* K 1 (Well, *Kupa* sira, Ether *Akasha* element point, sedation point. Sira related to Vata with the Well (Wind) sira of the Urinary Bladder channel)

Part of Talahridaya marma

Location: The point is located in the sole of the foot, in the depression when the foot is flexed, is located in the anterior third of the line between the base of the 2nd toe and heel of the foot. Between the 2nd and 3rd metatarsals.

Indications: Loss of consciousness, vertex pain, dizziness, blurred vision, sore throat, hoarseness, dry tongue, epistaxis, dysuria, difficult urination, sore neck and back, stabbing pain in the genitals, infantile seizure, pain and feverish sensation in the soles of the feet.

Talahridaya Marma Therapy: Stimulates kidneys (*Vata*).

Puncture: The needle is inserted perpendicularly to 0.3 - ½ anguli depth. Can be treated with *agnikarma*.

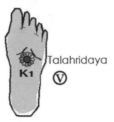

Fig. 28.

K 2 (Spring, *Sara* sira, Fire *Tejas* element point. Sira related to Pitta with the Spring (Water) sira of the Urinary Bladder channel)

Location: The point is located in the depression in the lower edge of the tuberosity of the navicular bone on the edge of the foot inferior and interior of the medial malleolus.

Indications: Irregular menstruation, uterine prolapse, perineal pruritus, abnormal seminal emission, inflammation and edema of the dorsum of the foot.

Puncture: The needle is inserted perpendicularly 0.3 anguli depth. Can be treated with *agnikarma*.

* K 3 (Stream, *Sarit* sira, and Base-*Mula* sira, Earth *Prithvi* element point)

Location: The point is located at the tip of the tip of the medial malleolus, in the depression between the medial malleolus and the calcaneal tendon.

Indications: Insomnia, impotence, disorders of the genito-urinary, asthma.

Puncture: The needle is inserted perpendicularly to 0.3 anguli depth. Can be treated with *agnikarma*.

* **K 4 (Bridge, *Setu* sira. Bridge point between Kidney and Urinary Bladder channels)**

   Location: The point is located in the insertion of the calcaneal tendon ligature in the posterior-inferior medial malleolus.

   Indications: Pain in the heel, asthma, hemoptysis, pain and stiffness in the lumbosacral region, dysuria.

   Puncture: The needle is inserted perpendicularly to 0.3 anguli depth. Can be treated with *agnikarma*.

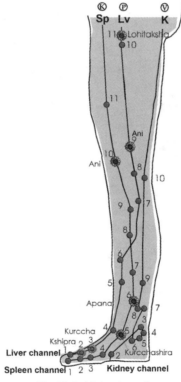

***Fig. 29.** Inside leg channels*

* **K 5 (Cleft, *Antara* sira)**

   Location: The point is located in the depression located anterior/ superior of the inner side of the tuberosity of the calcaneus, 1 anguli directly under K 3.

   Indications: Blurred vision, dysuria, abdominal pain, female disorders such as prolapse of the uterus, amenorrhea, irregular menstruation and dysmenorrhea.

   Puncture: The needle is inserted perpendicularly to 0.4 anguli depth. Can be treated with *agnikarma*.

* K 6

Location: The point is located in the depression, at a distance of 1 anguli below the medial malleolus.

Indications: Insomnia, epilepsy, sore throat, female disorders including uterine prolapse, perineal pruritus and irregular menstruation, hernia, frequent and weak urination.

Puncture: The needle is inserted perpendicularly to 0.3 - ½ anguli depth. Can be treated with *agnikarma*.

* K 7 (River, *Dhuni* sira, Air / Wind *Vayu* element point, tonification point. Sira related to Vata)

Location: The point is located 2 angulis above K 3 and 1 anguli below the malleolus.

Indications: Spontaneous night sweat, dry throat, weakness and paralysis of the legs.

Puncture: The needle is inserted perpendicularly to 0.3 - ½ anguli depth. Can be treated with *agnikarma*.

K 8

Location: The point is located at a distance of ½ anguli below K 7, at the trailing edge of the tibia.

Indications: Uterine prolapse, uterine bleeding, pain and swelling of the testicles, groin pain, lower abdominal pain, bloody diarrhea, urination and defecation difficulty.

Puncture: The needle is inserted perpendicularly to 0.4 anguli depth. Can be treated with *agnikarma*.

K 9

Location: The point is located in the inside of the calf muscles, 5 angulis above the tip of the medial malleolus.

Indications: Mental disorders, pain on the inside of the leg.

Puncture: The needle is inserted perpendicularly to ½ -0.8 anguli depth. Can be treated with *agnikarma*.

K 10 (Sea, *Samudra* sira, Water *Jala* element point. Sira related to Kapha along with the Sea (Earth) sira of the Urinary Bladder channel. Sira which controls Sleshaka Kapha.)

Location: The point is located at the popliteal crease at the level of the medial border of the semitendinous.

Indications: Hair loss, swelling and fullness of the lower abdomen, difficult urination, dark urine, impotence, hernia, overall itching, bleeding, disorders of the knees.

Puncture: The needle is inserted perpendicularly to 0.8 - 1 anguli depth. Can be treated with *agnikarma*.

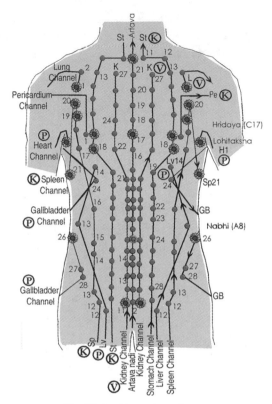

Fig. 30. *Front torso channels*

* K 11
Vitapa marma
Location: The point is located at a distance of ½ anguli sideways of C2, at the upper edge of the symphysis pubis.

Indications: Impotence, abnormal seminal emission, pain of the genitals, urinary retention.

Vitapa Marma Therapy: Impotence, retention of urine, painful external genital and seminal emission. Affects the muscle tone in the lower abdomen.

Puncture: The needle is inserted perpendicularly to ½ -0.8 anguli depth. Can be treated with *agnikarma*.

K 12
Location: The point is located at a distance of ½ anguli outwards of C 3, approximately at 4 angulis below the navel.

Indications: Disorders of the genitals.

Puncture: The needle is inserted perpendicularly to ½ - 1 anguli depth. Can be treated with *agnikarma*.

K 13

Location: The point is located at a distance of ½ anguli outside the point C 4.
Indications: Irregular menstruation.
Puncture: The needle is inserted perpendicularly to ½ - 1 anguli depth. Can be treated with *agnikarma*.

K 14

Location: The point is located at a distance of ½ anguli outside the point C5.
Indications: Postpartum abdominal pain, irregular menstruation, uterine bleeding.
Puncture: The needle is inserted perpendicularly to ½ - 1 anguli depth. Can be treated with *agnikarma*.

K 15

Location: The point is located at a distance of ½ anguli outside the point C 7.
Indications: Constipation, lower abdominal pain, irregular menstruation.
Puncture: The needle is inserted perpendicularly to ½ - 1 anguli depth. Can be treated with *agnikarma*.

K 16

Location: The point is located at a distance of ½ anguli outside the center of the navel.
Indications: Constipation, bloating and abdominal pain, vomiting.
Puncture: The needle is inserted perpendicularly to ½ - 1 anguli depth. Can be treated with *agnikarma*.

K 17

Location: The point is located at a distance of ½ anguli outside the point C 10.
Indications: Constipation, abdominal distention, pain and diarrhea.
Puncture: The needle is inserted perpendicularly to ½ - 1 anguli depth. Can be treated with *agnikarma*.

K 18

Location: The point is located at a distance of ½ anguli outside the point C 11.
Indications: Constipation, abdominal pain (postpartum) vomiting.
Puncture: The needle is inserted perpendicularly to ½ - 1 anguli depth. Can be treated with *agnikarma*.

K 19

Location: The point is located at a distance of ½ anguli outside the point C 12.
Indications: Disorders of the abdomen.
Puncture: The needle is inserted perpendicularly to ½ - 1 anguli depth. Can be treated with *agnikarma*.

K 20

Location: The point is located at a distance of ½ anguli outside the point C 13.
Indications: Disorders of the abdomen with vomiting, diarrhea.
Puncture: The needle is inserted perpendicularly to ½ - 1 anguli depth. Can be treated with *agnikarma*.

K 21

Location: The point is located at a distance of ½ anguli outside the point C 14.
Indications: Disorders of the abdomen with vomiting, diarrhea.
Puncture: The needle is inserted perpendicularly to 0.3 - 0.7 anguli depth. Can be treated with *agnikarma*.

K 22

Location: The point is located at a distance of 2 angulis outside the Artava channel (C) in the fifth intercostal space.
Indications: Cough and asthma.
Puncture: The needle is inserted obliquely to 0.3 - ½ anguli depth. Can be treated with *agnikarma*.

K 23

Location: The point is located at a distance of 2 angulis outside the Artava channel (C) in the fourth intercostal space.
Indications: Mastitis, chest tightness and cough, asthma.
Puncture: The needle is inserted obliquely to 0.3 - ½ anguli depth. Can be treated with *agnikarma*.

K 24

Location: The point is located at a distance of 2 angulis outside the Artava channel (C) in the third intercostal space.
Indications: Mastitis, chest tightness and cough, asthma.
Puncture: The needle is inserted obliquely to 0.3 - ½ anguli depth. Can be treated with *agnikarma*.

K 25

Location: The point is located at a distance of 2 angulis outside the Artava channel (C) in the second intercostal space.
Indications: Chest pain, asthma, coughs.
Puncture: The needle is inserted obliquely to 0.3 - ½ anguli depth. Can be treated with *agnikarma*.

K 26

Location: The point is located at a distance of 2 angulis outside the Artava channel (C) in the first intercostal space.
Indications: Pressure in the chest and hypochondrium, asthma.
Puncture: The needle is inserted obliquely to 0.3 - ½ anguli depth. Can be treated with *agnikarma*.

K 27

Location: The point is located at a distance of 2 angulis outside the Artava channel (C) in the depression on the border of the clavicle.
Indications: Chest pain, tightness and fullness in the chest, dyspnoea, asthma.
Puncture: The needle is inserted perpendicularly to 0.3 anguli depth. Can be treated with *agnikarma*.

Dhamanis of PITTA (*SECONDARY*) - Leg

GALLBLADDER CHANNEL (Figures 26, 27, 30 and 31)

Channel Name: Pittashaya Dhamani
  Organ: Gall Bladder *Pittashaya*
  Element: Ether *Akasha*
  Dosha: Pitta (Secondary)
  Energy Peak Hours: 12am (between 11pm-1am)
  Channel location: External side of both legs
  Number of Siras: 44
  Energy Flow: Descending (Ashaya dhamani) *centrifugal*. Transmits Prana flow to its related dosha- Pitta- Liver channel which itself has an ascending flow. The Gallbladder receives the flow of Prana from the previous channel, Tridosha channel, of Kapha dosha.

Siras of the Pittashaya Dhamani-Gallbladder

Indications and location of the points of Pittashaya dhamani (GB):
* *Demonstrates siras used often.*

GB 44 (Well, *Kupa* sira, Wind / Air *Vayu* element point. Sira related to Vata with the Well (Ether) sira of the Liver channel)
   Location: The point is located at a distance of 0.1 anguli posterior to the nail on the outer side of the fourth toe.
   Indications: Sleep disorders, fever, deafness, migraine, eye pain, pain in the hypochondrium.
   Puncture: The needle is inserted obliquely to 0.1-0.2 anguli depth. Can be treated with *agnikarma*.

GB 43 (Spring, *Sara* sira, Water *Jala* element point, tonification point. Sira related to Pitta with the Spring (Fire) sira of the Liver channel. (Pitta = Fire and Water)
   Location: The point is located in the anterior part of the fourth and fifth metatarsophalangeal joint, at the margin of the angle between the fourth and fifth toes.
   Indications: Febrile diseases, blurred vision, pain in the cheeks and in the outer corner of eye, tinnitus, submandibular and upper quadrant pain.
   Puncture: The needle is inserted obliquely upwards to 0.2 to 0.3 anguli depth. Can be treated with *agnikarma*.

* GB 42

Part of Pada Kurccha Marma (with Lv 3)
   Location: The point is located in the inside of the digital extensor tendon of the foot between the fourth and fifth metatarsal.
   Indications: Flushing and edema of the rear of foot, eye pain, red eyes, distended breasts, edema in the axillary region, hypertension.
   Pada Kurccha Marma Therapy: Hypertension, jaundice, uterine bleeding.
   Puncture: The needle is inserted perpendicularly to 0.3 - 0.4 anguli depth. Can be treated with *agnikarma*.

* GB 41 (Stream, *Sarit* sira, Ether *Akasha* element point. Sira related to Vata)
   Location: The point is located in a depression immediately and distal to the joint at the base of the fourth and fifth metatarsal.
   Indications: Stagnation of Prana in the head region (cephaleas, conjunctivitis, deafness), blurred vision, eye redness, grittiness in the eye, pain in the outer corner of eye, vertigo, deafness and tinnitus, foot pain, ear disorders and breast cancer.
   Puncture: The needle is inserted perpendicularly to 0.3 - ½ anguli depth. Can be treated with *agnikarma*.

* **GB 40 (Base, *Mula* sira. Point directly related to the Gallbladder)**
  Location: The point is located in the depression at the edge above the lateral malleolus.
  Indications: Pain and swelling in the neck, chest and hypochondrium and ankle, swelling of the axillary region, malaria, blurred vision, vomiting, acid regurgitation, weakness and pain in the legs.
  Puncture The needle is inserted perpendicularly to 0.3 - ½ anguli depth. Can be treated with *agnikarma*.

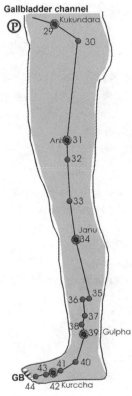

Fig. 31. *Outside leg channel*

* **GB 39 (the meeting point of bone)**

Part of Gulpha Marma (with UB 59)
  Location: The point is located in the depression, 3 angulis above the end of the lateral malleolus.
  Indications: Disorders of the bone / marrow, pain and paralysis of legs and neck pain.
  Gulpha Marma Therapy: Treatment of paralysis of the leg and pain (especially in the ankle joint).
  Puncture: The needle is inserted perpendicularly to 0.4 - ½ anguli depth. Can be treated with *agnikarma*.

* GB 38 (River, *Dhuni* sira, Fire *Tejas* element point, sedation point. Sira related to Pitta)

    Location: The point is located at a distance of 4 angulis a little anterior and above the tip of the lateral malleolus.

    Indications: Arthritis of knee, headache, feeling of heat in the head as if on fire, pain in the outer corner of eye, pain in the supraclavicular fossa and axillary region, malaria, blockages along the dhamani, scrofula, pain in throat, chest, upper quadrant and on the outside of the legs.

    Puncture: The needle is inserted perpendicularly to ½ -0.7 anguli depth. Can be treated with *agnikarma*.

* GB 37 (Bridge, *Setu* sira. Bridge point between Gallbladder and Liver channels)

    Location: The point is located at the anterior border of the fibula, a distance of 5 angulis above the tip of the lateral malleolus.

    Indications: Eye disorders (myopia, blurred vision, poor night vision), pain in the knees, legs and breasts.

    Puncture: The needle is inserted perpendicularly to 0.7 - 1 anguli depth. Can be treated with *agnikarma*.

* GB 36 (Cleft, *Antara* sira)

    Location: The point is located at the anterior border of the fibula, a distance of 7 angulis above the tip of the lateral malleolus.

    Indications: Headaches, tingling in calves, pain and stiffness in neck, chest and hypochondrium.

    Puncture: The needle is inserted perpendicularly to ½ -0.8 anguli depth. Can be treated with *agnikarma*.

GB 35

    Location: The point is located level and slightly above the GB 36 in the posterior border of the fibula.

    Indications: Palpitations, panic, mania, tightness in the chest, pain and weakness in hips, knees and legs.

    Puncture: The needle is inserted perpendicularly to ½ -0.8 anguli depth. Can be treated with *agnikarma*.

* GB 34 (Sea, *Samudra* sira, Earth *Prithvi* element point. Sira related to Kapha with the Sea (Water) sira of the Liver channel)

It is part of Janu Marma (with UB40 and St 35)

    Location: The point is located in the depression that lies anterior and below the fibular head.

    Indications: Mental disorders, arterial hypertension, dizziness, vomiting, epilepsy, gallbladder disease, bitter taste in the mouth, pain, stiffness and contracture of the muscles and tendons of the legs.

    Janu Marma Therapy: Treats pain in leg and lower back, including the hip joint.

    Puncture: The needle is inserted perpendicularly to 0.8 - 1.2 anguli depth. Can be treated with *agnikarma*.

GB 33

    Location: The point is located in the depression lateral to the knee joint and 3 angulis above GB 34.

    Indications: Numbness in the legs, pain and edema in knees.

    Puncture: The needle is inserted perpendicularly to ½ anguli depth.

GB 32

    Location: The point is located at a distance of 5 angulis above the popliteal transverse crease.

    Indications: Numbness, pain and leg weakness, hemiplegia, muscle atrophy.

    Puncture: The needle is inserted perpendicularly to ½ -0.8 anguli depth. Can be treated with *agnikarma*.

* GB 31

Forms part of lower limb Ani Marma (with St 33, -Sp 10 and Lv 9 and on the inside of leg)

    Location: The point is located at a distance of 7 angulis above the knee crease, on the outer thigh.

    Indications: Paralysis in children, movement disorders and leg pain, hemiplegia, sciatica, muscular atrophy.

    Ani Marma Therapy: Controls muscle tone.

    Puncture: The needle is inserted perpendicularly to 0.7 - 1.2 anguli depth. Can be treated with *agnikarma*.

* GB 30
Location: The point is located sideways and a little inferior than UB 54, near the greater trochanter.
Indications: Lumbago, sciatica, hemiplegia, pain in the hip region, muscular atrophy, motor disorders, pain and weakness of legs (difficulty to flex or extend).
Puncture: The needle is inserted perpendicularly to 1 ½ -2.5 angulis depth. Can be treated with *agnikarma*.

* GB 29 (Sira controlling Shukravaha Srotas and Mutravaha Srotas)
Kukundara Marma
Location: The point is located midway between the greater trochanter and anterior superior iliac spine.
Indications: Paralysis, pain in the back and legs.
Kukundara Marma Therapy: Controls Raktavaha srotas and the formation of blood. To stimulate Rasavaha srotas massage using patchouli oil.
Puncture: The needle is inserted perpendicularly to ½ - 1 anguli depth. Can be treated with *agnikarma*.

GB 28
Location: The point is located at a distance of ½ anguli antero-inferior of the point GB 27.
Indications: Lumbago, prolapse of the uterus, pain in the hip joint, leucorrhea, lower abdominal pain.
Puncture: The needle is inserted perpendicularly to ½ - 1 anguli depth. Can be treated with *agnikarma*.

GB 27
Location: The point is located at a distance of 3 angulis below the level of the navel, above the anterior superior iliac spine (½ anguli away).
Indications: Lumbago and pain in the hip joint, hernia, leucorrhea.
Puncture: The needle is inserted perpendicularly to ½ - 1 anguli depth. Can be treated with *agnikarma*.

* GB 26
Part of Parshva Sandhi Marma
Location: The point is located at the level of the navel, directly below the free end of the eleventh rib.
Indications: Lumbago, upper quadrant pain, prolapsed uterus, irregular menstruation, leucorrhea, amenorrhea, hernia.
Therapy of Parshva Sandhi Marma: Assists circulation, "controls the second chakra, ovaries and adrenal glands." (Ranade, et al, 1999, 72)
Puncture: The needle is inserted perpendicularly to ½ - 1 anguli depth. Can be treated with *agnikarma*.

* **GB 25 (Front point of the Kidney and Medavaha Srotas)**
  Location: The point is located in the lower edge of the free end of the twelfth rib.
  Indications: Lumbago, nephritis, difficult urination and dark urine, pain affecting the back and hypochondrium, rumbling, chronic diarrhea, abdominal distension.
  Puncture: The needle is inserted perpendicularly to 0.3 - ½ anguli depth. Can be treated with *agnikarma*.

* **GB 24 (Front point of the Gallbladder and Raktavaha Srotas)**
  Location: The point is located inferior to the nipple, between the seventh and eighth ribs.
  Indications: Hepatitis, cholecystitis, nausea and vomiting, acid regurgitation, bitter mouth, frequent sighing, hiccups, sadness, difficulty speaking, weakness, jaundice due to obstruction, lithiasis.
  Puncture: The needle is inserted obliquely to 0.3 - ½ anguli depth. Can be treated with *agnikarma*.

GB 23
  Location: The point is located almost at the level of the nipples, a distance of 1 anguli below point GB 22.
  Indications: Asthma and tightness in the chest.
  Puncture: The needle is inserted obliquely to 0.3 - ½ anguli depth. Can be treated with *agnikarma*.

GB 22
  Location: The point is located at a distance of 3 angulis below the armpit, in the mid-axillary line.
  Indications: Pain and edema in the axillary region and hypochondrium.
  Puncture: The needle is inserted obliquely to 0.3 - ½ anguli depth. Can be treated with *agnikarma*.

* **GB 21**
Part of Amsa Marma
  Location: The point is located between the midpoint of the clavicle and the top of the scapula, between GB 14 and the acromion.
  Indications: Disorders of the thyroid and endocrine system, hypogalactia, mastitis, shoulder pain, neck and back, difficult childbirth, stroke, vomiting, nausea, shortness of breath.
  Amsa Marma Therapy: Stimulates Throat chakra, thyroid and endocrine system.
  Puncture: The needle is inserted perpendicularly to ½ anguli depth. Can be treated with *agnikarma*.

* GB 20
Part of Matrika Marma (with GB 15, TD 16, SI 17 and C 23)
  Location: The point is located in the medial depression of the mastoid process in the back of the neck, 1 anguli from hairline, between the middle and the lower edge of the mastoid bone.
  Indications: Flu, colds, nasal obstruction, headache, dizziness, vertigo, red eyes and eye pain, loss of vision, febrile diseases without sweating, tearing, runny nose, difficulty in swallowing, pain in the neck, shoulder and back.
  Matrika Marma Therapy: Enhances circulation in the head. Controls majjavaha srotas (channels of the nervous system).
  Puncture: The needle is inserted perpendicularly to ½ - 1 anguli depth, with the tip of the needle towards the tip of the nose. Can be treated with *agnikarma*.

GB 19
  Location: The point is located in the depression between the upper and eidomastoid esternocl muscle m. trapezius, level with G 17 at the outer side of the occipital protuberance, halfway between this and the top edge of the mastoid bone.
  Indications: Pain and stiffness in neck and head.
  Puncture: The needle is inserted horizontally to 0.3 - ½ anguli depth pointing down. Can be treated with *agnikarma*.

GB 18
  Location: The point is located at a distance of 2.25 angulis from the midline (G) and 1 ½ anguli posterior to point GB 17.
  Indications: Epistaxis, rhinorrhea, headache.
  Puncture: The needle is inserted horizontally to 0.3 - ½ anguli depth pointing down. Can be treated with *agnikarma*.

GB 17
  Location: The point is located at a distance of 2.25 angulis from the midline (G) and 1 ½ anguli posterior to point GB 16.
  Indications: Blurred vision, migraine.
  Puncture: The needle is inserted horizontally to 0.3 - ½ anguli depth pointing backwards. Can be treated with *agnikarma*.

GB 16
  Location: The point is located at a distance of 1 ½ anguli posterior to GB15 point between this point and GB20.
  Indications: Blurred vision headache, red eyes and eye pain.
  Puncture: The needle is inserted horizontally to 0.3 - ½ anguli depth pointing back. Can be treated with *agnikarma*.

* GB 15
Part of Shringataka Marma (with UB 5, G 22, G 23)
Location: The point is located between points G 24 and St 8, is directly above the point GB 14.

Indications: Blurred vision, headache, lacrimation, nasal obstruction, sore eye.

Shringataka Marma Therapy: Stimulates the nervous system and soothes the eyes, ears, nose and tongue.

Puncture: The needle is inserted horizontally to 0.3 - ½ anguli depth pointing up. Can be treated with *agnikarma*.

* GB 14
Part of Avarta Marma
Location: The point is located at a distance of 1 anguli above the midpoint of the eyebrow.

Indications: Disorders of sight (including glaucoma, blurred vision) and sinus headache, facial paralysis.

Avarta Marma Therapy: Diseases of vision, sinusitis (frontal) and temporal headaches.

Puncture: The needle is inserted horizontally to 0.3 - ½ anguli depth pointing down. Can be treated with *agnikarma*.

GB13
Location: The point is located at a distance of 3 angulis outside the midline of the body at the level of G 24.

Indications: Mental disorders, epilepsy, headache, blurred vision.

Puncture: The needle is inserted horizontally to 0.3 - ½ anguli depth pointing backwards. Can be treated with *agnikarma*.

GB 12
Location: The point is located in the depression that exists at the bottom and back of the mastoid process.

Indications: Insomnia, facial paralysis, toothache, headache.

Puncture: The needle is inserted obliquely pointing down to 0.3 - ½ anguli depth. Can be treated with **agnikarma**.

GB 11
Location: The point is located between GB 10 and GB 12, above and posterior to the mastoid process.

Indications: Deafness, headache, ear and neck pain.

Puncture: The needle is inserted horizontally to 0.3 anguli depth. Can be treated with *agnikarma*.

GB 10

Location: The point is located between points GB 9 and GB 11, 1 anguli posterior and oblique to GB 8.

Indications: Deafness, headache.

Puncture: The needle is inserted horizontally to 0.3 anguli depth. Can be treated with *agnikarma*.

GB 9

Location: The point is located at a distance of ½ anguli obliquely and posterior to GB 8 in the anterior part to the ear.

Indications: Depression, headache, gingivitis.

Puncture: The needle is inserted horizontally.

GB 8

Location: The point is located at a distance of 1 ½ anguli from the hairline directly above the top of the ear.

Indications: Migraine (Pitta-type), vertigo, nausea, vomiting and seizures in children.

Puncture: The needle is inserted horizontally to 0.3 - ½ anguli depth. Can be treated with *agnikarma*.

GB 7

Location: The point is located a finger width to point TD 20 and is within the hairline on the anterior part of the top of the ear.

Indications: Pitta type pain in head (temporal area), contraction of m. masseter and edema of the cheeks.

Puncture: The needle is inserted horizontally to 0.2 -0.3 anguli depth pointing backwards. Can be treated with *agnikarma*.

GB 6

Location: The point is located between points GB 5 and GB 7 on the hairline, below the temporal angle.

Indications: Pitta headache, eye pain.

Puncture: The needle is inserted horizontally to 0.2 - 0.3 anguli depth pointing back. Can be treated with *agnikarma*.

GB 5

Location: The point is located between points St 8 and GB 7, within the hairline in the temporal region.

Indications: Pitta headache, eye pain.

Puncture: The needle is inserted horizontally to 0.3 - ½ anguli depth. Can be treated with *agnikarma*.

* GB 4
Part of Shringataka Marma (with UB 4, St 8)
   Location: The point is located between points St 8 and GB 5, within the hairline in the temporal region.
   Indications: Pitta headache, eye pain, blurred vision.
   Shringataka Marma Therapy: Stimulates the nervous system and soothes the eyes, ears, nose and tongue.
   Puncture: The needle is inserted horizontally to 0.3 - ½ anguli depth. Can be treated with *agnikarma*.

GB 3
   Location: The point is located in the depression directly above the point St 7 in front of the ear, in the upper edge of the zygomatic arch.
   Indications: Pitta headache, facial paralysis, deafness, toothache.
   Puncture: The needle is inserted perpendicularly to 0.3 anguli depth. Deep insertions are contraindicated. Can be treated with *agnikarma*.

GB 2
   Location: The point is located in depression directly below the point SI 19 below the mandibular condyloid process.
   Indications: Vertigo with sensation of falling, chronic ear infections, tinnitus, deafness, ear pain, dental pain, dislocation and arthritis of the jaw, cheek pain, difficulty chewing, facial paralysis.
   Puncture: The needle is inserted perpendicularly to ½ -0.7 anguli depth. Can be treated with *agnikarma*.

* GB 1
Part of Apanga Marma (with TD 23)
   Location: The point is located in the depression on the outside of the eye socket.
   Indications:, Progressive loss of vision, blurred vision, night blindness, eye pain, photophobia, eyelid twitching, eyes red and watery, headache.
   Apanga Marma Therapy: Reduces nervous stress and can treat defective vision.
   Puncture: The needle is inserted horizontally to 0.2 anguli depth. Can be treated with *agnikarma*.

LIVER CHANNEL (Figures 29 and 30) *Pitta* - Leg

Channel Name: Yakrt Dhamani
  Organ: Liver *Yakrt*
  Element: Ether
  Dosha: Pitta (Secondary)
  Energy Peak Hours: 2:00 a.m. (1-3 am)
  Channel location: Inside of both legs
  Number of Siras: 14
  Energy Flow: Ascending (Dhatu dhamani) *centripetal*. Transmits Pranic flow to the next dosha - Vata-the Lung channel which itself has a descending flow. The Liver receives the flow of Prana from the previous channel, the Gallbladder channel of its related dosha-Pitta.

Siras of Yakrt Dhamani-Liver

Indications and location of the points of Yakrt dhamani (Lv):
Demonstrates siras used often.

Lv 1 (Well, *Kupa* sira, Ether *Akasha* element point. Sira related to Vata, with the Well (Air) sira of the Urinary Bladder Channel). BhutaAgni of Ether)
  Location: The point is located near the corner or inner angle of the nail of the big toe.
  Indications: Psychic alterations, drowsiness wanting to close the eyes, vertigo, sighs, abdominal pain and swelling, edema and pain of the external genitalia, uterine prolapse, hernia, uterine bleeding, urinary difficulty, enuresis.
  Puncture: The needle is inserted obliquely to 0.1-0.2 anguli depth. Can be treated with *agnikarma*.

Lv 2 (Spring, *Sara* sira, Fire *Tejas* element point, sedation point. Sira related to Pitta along with the Spring (Water) sira of the Urinary Bladder channel. Sira which controls Ranjaka Pitta and Svedavaha Srotas. BhutaAgni of Fire)

Part of Pada Kshipra Marma

Location: The point is located at the joint of the big toe and the second toe.

Indications: Insomnia, headache, dizziness, menorrhagia, urethritis, enuresis, urinary retention, hernia, deviation of the mouth, feeling of constriction in the throat, flushing, cough, asthma, edema, eye pain, blurred vision, pain in hypochondrium, pain and swelling of the knee, epilepsy, convulsions, tremors.

Pada Kshipra Marma Therapy: Swelling, redness and pain in the eyes and the toes. "Indications: pain, bleeding and seizures." (Joshi, et al, 2005, 109)

Puncture: The needle is inserted obliquely to ½ anguli depth. Can be treated with *agnikarma*.

* Lv 3 (Stream, *Sarit* sira, Base-*Mula* sira, Earth *Prithvi* element point, Kapha. Sira related to Alochaka Pitta and Svedavaha Srotas. BhutaAgni of Earth)

Part of Pada Kurccha Marma (with GB 42).

Location: The point is located in the depression, a little distal from the joint of the first and second metatarsals.

Indications: Insomnia, epilepsy, headache, dizziness, eye inflammation, blurred vision, dry and sore throat, feeling of fullness in the hypochondrium, bolus hystericum, abdominal pain, bowel sounds, nausea and vomiting, anorexia, diarrhea, constipation, jaundice, genital pain, metrorrhagia, amenorrhea, hernia, enuresis, urinary retention, back pain, pain in the front of the medial malleolus, deviation of the mouth, childhood seizure.

Pada Kurccha Marma Therapy: Hypertension pressure, jaundice, uterine bleeding.

Puncture: The needle is inserted perpendicularly to ½ anguli depth. Can be treated with *agnikarma*.

Lv 4 (River, *Dhuni* sira, Air / Wind *Vayu* element point. Sira related to Vata. BhutaAgni of Wind/Air)

Location: The point is located in the depression, at a distance of 1 anguli anterior to the medial malleolus, between Sp 5 and St 41.

Indications: Spermatorrhea, urinary retention, external genital pain, hernia, periumbilical pain, ankle pain difficulty to walk.

Puncture: The needle is inserted perpendicularly to 0.3 - ½ anguli depth. Can be treated with *agnikarma*.

Lv 5 (Bridge, *Setu* sira. Bridge point between Liver and Gallbladder channels)

Location: The point is located at a distance of 5 angulis above the tip of the medial malleolus.

Indications: Hernia, all kinds of sexual alterations (spermatorrhea, premature ejaculation, impotence), orchitis, vaginal itching, leucorrhoea, irregular menstruation, metrorrhagia and hypermetrorrhea, dysuria, enuresis, pain in legs.

Puncture: The needle is inserted horizontally to 0.3 - ½ anguli depth to the back. Can be treated with *agnikarma*.

* Lv 6 (Cleft, *Antara* sira)

Location: The point is located at a distance of 7 angulis above the tip of the medial malleolus.

Indications: Hernia, uterine bleeding, jaundice, abdominal pain, pain in external genitalia, arthritis in leg that makes standing difficult, heat in the sole of the foot.

Puncture: The needle is inserted horizontally to 0.3 - ½ anguli depth. Can be treated with *agnikarma*.

Lv 7

Location: The point is located at a distance of 1 anguli postero - inferior to the medial condyle of the tibia.

Indications: Pain on the inside of the knees.

Puncture: The needle is inserted perpendicularly to 0.4-0.6 anguli depth. Can be treated with *agnikarma*.

* Lv 8 (Sea, *Samudra* sira, Water *Jala* element point, tonification point. Sira related to Kapha along with the Sea (Earth) sira of the Gall Bladder channel. BhutaAgni of Water)

Location: The point is located at the end of the medial transverse crease of the knee.

Indications: Impotence, mania, uterine prolapse, pain in lower abdomen, difficulty urinating, urinary retention, pruritus vulvae, spermatorrhea, pain on the inside of the knee and leg pain and itching of external genitalia, heat in the body without sweat.

Puncture: The needle is inserted perpendicularly to ½ - 1 anguli depth. Can be treated with *agnikarma*.

* Lv 9

Part of Ani Marma (with UB 10, in addition to GB 31 and St33 on the outside)

Location: The point is located at a distance of 4 angulis above the medial epicondyle of the femur (Lv 8).

Indications: Muscle disorders, dysuria, irregular menstruation, pain in the lumbosacral region and abdomen.

Ani Marma Therapy: Controls muscle tone.

Puncture: The needle is inserted perpendicularly to 0.6-0.7 anguli depth. Can be treated with *agnikarma*.

Lv 10

Location: The point is located at a distance of 3 angulis below the point St 30.

Indications: Retention of urine, lower abdominal distension.

Puncture: The needle is inserted perpendicularly to ½ - 1 anguli depth. Can be treated with *agnikarma*.

* Lv 11

Part of Lohitaksha Marma (with H 1 in axilla)

Location: The point is located at a distance of 2 angulis below the point St 30.

Indications: Pain in the thighs and legs, irregular menstruation.

Lohitaksha Marma Therapy: Assists circulation and pain in the extremities. Controls Rasavaha Srotas.

Puncture: The needle is inserted perpendicularly to ½ - 1 anguli depth. Can be treated with *agnikarma*.

Lv 12

Location: The point is located at a distance of 2 ½ angulis outside the Artava channel (C) in the inguinal groove.

Indications: Hernia, external genital pain.

Puncture: The needle is inserted perpendicularly to ½ - 1 anguli depth. Can be treated with *agnikarma*.

* Lv 13 (Front point of the Spleen and of Udakavaha Srotas)

Location: The point is located inferior to the free end of the eleventh floating rib.

Indications: Nervousness, anorexia, vomiting, bloating, borborygmus, diarrhea, indigestion, hepatitis, jaundice, emaciation, epigastric pain and vomiting, upper quadrant pain and intercostal neuralgia, dyspnoea, fatigue of the four limbs, thoracolumbar pain with cold feeling that prevents rotation.

Puncture: Insert the needle perpendicularly to 0.8 - 1 anguli depth. Can be treated with *agnikarma*.

* **Lv 14 (Front point of the Liver and Raktavaha Srotas)**
  Location: The point is located in the sixth intercostal space on the chest, two ribs below the nipple.
  Indications: Nervous depression, anorexia, vomiting, chest pain, upper quadrant pain, breast disorders, abdominal pain, chest tightness, nervousness, cough and dyspnoea, hiccups, acid regurgitation.
  Puncture: The needle is inserted obliquely to 0.3 anguli depth. Can be treated with *agnikarma*.

Dhamanis of KAPHA (*SECONDARY*) - Arm

PERICARDIUM CHANNEL (Figures 22 and 30)

Channel Name: Talahridaya Dhamani
  Organ: Pericardium *Talahridaya*
  Element: Water (+) *Jala*
  Dosha: Kapha (Secondary)
  Peak Hours Energy: 8pm (between 7-9 pm)
  Channel location: Interior of both arms
  Number of Siras: 9
  Energy Flow: Descending (Ashaya dhamani) *centrifugal*. Transmits Pranic flow to its related dosha-Kapha-related the Tridosha channel which itself has an ascending flow. The Pericardium channel receives the flow of Prana from the previous channel, the Kidney channel of the Vata dosha.

Siras of Talahridaya Dhamani-Pericardium
  Indications and location of the points of Talahridaya dhamani (P):
  * *Demonstrates siras used often.*

P 9 (Well, *Kupa* sira, Ether *Akasha* element point, tonification point. Sira related to Vata with the Well (Wind/Air) sira of the 3D channel)
  Location: The point is located in the center of the tip of the middle finger of the hand.
  Indications: Syncope (loss of consciousness), febrile diseases, irritability, chest pain, aphasia with stiffness of the tongue, heat stroke, childhood seizure, heat in the palms.
  Puncture: The needle is inserted perpendicularly to 0.3 - ½ anguli depth. Can be treated with *agnikarma*.

* P 8 (Spring, *Sara* sira, Fire *Tejas* element point, sira related to Pitta with the Spring (Water) sira of the 3D Tridosha channel. Sira which controls Sadhaka Pitta, Pranavayu and PranaVaha Srotas)

Part of Talahridaya Marma

Location: The point is located in the palm of the hand between the second and third metacarpals.

Indications: Epilepsy, mental disorders, vomiting, chest pain, stomatitis, halitosis, fungal infections of the hand and foot.

Puncture: The needle is inserted perpendicularly to 0.3 - ½ anguli depth. Can be treated with *agnikarma*.

* P 7 (Stream, *Sarit* sira, Earth *Prithvi* element point, Base-*Mula* sira, Kapha, sedation point. Sira related to Sadhaka Pitta)

Location: The point lies in depression in the middle of the transverse crease of the wrist.

Indications: Mental disorders, epilepsy, panic, palpitation, chest pain and chest and hypochondrium, stomach pain, vomiting, disorders of the wrist.

Puncture: The needle is inserted perpendicularly to 0.3 - ½ anguli depth. Can be treated with *agnikarma*.

* P 6 (Bridge, *Setu* sira). Bridge point between Pericardium and Tridosha channels. Sira which controls Udana vayu.)

Udana sira

Location: The point is located at a distance of 2 angulis proximal to transverse wrist crease and P 7.

Indications: Mental disorders, epilepsy, palpitation, febrile diseases and malaria, chest pain, stomach pain, vomiting, contraction of elbow and arm. Point for anesthesia for surgery of the thyroid and heart.

Puncture: The needle is inserted perpendicularly to ½ - 1 anguli depth. Can be treated with *agnikarma*.

* P 5 (River, *Dhuni* sira, Air/Wind *Vayu* element point. Sira related to Vata)

Location: The point is located at a distance of 3 angulis proximal to transverse wrist crease.

Indications: Mental disorders, epilepsy, irritability, malaria, palpitation, febrile diseases, precordial pain, stomach pain, vomiting, swelling in the armpit, twitch or contraction of the elbow, arm pain.

Puncture: The needle is inserted perpendicularly to ½ - 1 anguli depth. Can be treated with *agnikarma*.

* P 4 (Cleft–*Antara* sira)
Part of Indrabasti Marma (with L 6 and TD 9)
  Location: The point is located at a distance of 5 angulis proximal to the transverse crease of the wrist, the line connecting P 3 and P 7.
  Indications: Palpitation and acute cardiac chest pain, hematemesis, epistaxis, boils.
  Indrabasti Marma Therapy: Stimulates Agni, the digestive 'Fire'.
  Puncture: The needle is inserted perpendicularly to ½ -0.8 anguli depth. Can be treated with *agnikarma*.

* **P 3 (Sea, *Samudra* sira, Water *Jala* element point. Sira related to Kapha along with the Sea (Earth) sira of the Tridosha 3D channel. Sira which controls Tarpaka Kapha and Pranavaha Srotas)**
  Location: The point is located at the transverse crease of the elbow joint on the side of the biceps tendon.
  Indications: Palpitation, anxiety, irritability, stomach pain, vomiting, febrile diseases in pain, chest pain, pain and upper limb tremor.
  Puncture: The needle is inserted perpendicularly to ½ -0.8 anguli depth. Can be treated with *agnikarma*.

* **P 2**
Part of Urvi Marma
  Location: The point is located between the two ends of m. biceps brachii, a distance of 2 angulis below the end of the anterior axillary crease.
  Indications: Cough, pain in chest, back and inside of the upper limbs, distention of hypochondrium.
  Puncture: The needle is inserted perpendicularly to ½ -0.7 anguli depth. Can be treated with *agnikarma*.

P 1
  Location: The point is located in the fourth intercostal space and a distance of 1 anguli from the nipple.
  Indications: Pain and edema in the axillary region, sensation of tightness in the chest.
  Puncture: The needle is inserted obliquely to 0.2 anguli depth carefully. Deep insertion is contraindicated in this sira. Can be treated with *agnikarma*.

TRIDOSHA CHANNEL (Figures 23, 26 and 27)
Kapha - Arm

Channel Name: Shleshmashay Dhamani
   Organ: Tridosha or 3D *Shleshmashay*
   Element: Water (+) *Jala*
   Dosha: Kapha (Secondary)
   Peak Hours Energy: 10pm (between 9-11 pm)
   Channel location: Exterior of both arms (center)
   Energy Flow: Ascending (Dhatu dhamani) *centripetal*. The channel Tridosha receives Pranic flow from the previous channel, the Pericardium Channel of its related dosha-Kapha. Transmits Prana flow to its next related dosha-Pitta- the Gallbladder channel that itself has a descending flow.

Siras of Shleshmashay dhamani-Tridosha

Indications and location of the points of Shleshmashay dhamani (TD - 3D): *Demonstrates siras siras used often.*

TD 1 (Well, *Kupa* sira, Wind/Air *Vayu* element point, Vata related point with the Well sira of the Pericardium channel)
   Location: The point is located at a distance of 0.1 anguli posterior to the corner of the nail, on the outer side of the ring finger.
   Indications: Febrile diseases, irritability, headache, red eyes, pharyngitis, stiffness of the tongue.
   Puncture: The needle is inserted obliquely to 0.1 anguli depth. Can be treated with *agnikarma*.

TD 2 (Spring, *Sara* sira, Water *Jala* element point, Pitta related point with the Spring sira of the Pericardium Channel. Sira which controls Sleshaka Kapha)
   Location: The point is located approximately at the edge of the corner of the ring and little fingers.
   Indications: Malaria, headache, deafness, red eyes, sore throat, pain in the arm.
   Puncture: The needle is inserted obliquely to 0.3-0.5 anguli depth into the space between the metacarpal bones. Can be treated with *agnikarma*.

* TD 3 (Stream, *Sarit* sira, Ether *Akasha* element point, tonification point.
Point related to Vata)
Part of Kurccha Marma (with LI 5)
  Location: The point is located in the depression in the back of the hand
  between the fourth and fifth metacarpals.
  Indications: Ear disorders (deafness, tinnitus) febrile illness, headache, red
  eyes, sore throat, pain in the elbow and arm, motor disorders of the fingers.
  Kurccha Marma Therapy: Treatment of the large intestine, pain.
  Puncture: The needle is inserted perpendicularly to 0.3 - ½ anguli depth.
  Can be treated with *agnikarma*.

* TD 4 (Base, *Mula* sira)
Part of Kurccha Shira Marma (with SI 5)
  Location: The point lies in the depression of the transverse crease of the
  dorsum of the wrist at the junction of the ulna and carpus.
  Indications: Malaria, deafness, pain in the wrist, shoulder and arm.
  Kurccha Shira Marma Therapy: Cardiac and pulmonary symptoms.
  Puncture: The needle is inserted perpendicularly to 0.3 anguli depth. Can
  be treated with *agnikarma*.

* TD 5 (Bridge, *Setu* sira. Bridge point between Tridosha and Pericardium
channels)

Part of Manibhanda Marma (with SI 5)
  Location: The point is located between the radius and ulna at a distance
  of 2 angulis above TD 4.
  Indications: Temporal headache (Pitta), febrile diseases, deafness, tinnitus,
  pain in the cheek and upper quadrant, arthritis of the arm, hand tremor,
  movement disorders of the elbow and arm pain of the fingers.
  Manibhanda Marma Therapy: Treats diseases of the wrist, carpal tunnel
  syndrome, cardiac pain and mental illness.
  Puncture: The needle is inserted perpendicularly to 0.7 to 1 anguli depth.
  Can be treated with *agnikarma*.

* TD 6 (River, *Dhuni* sira, Fire *Tejas* element point. Sira related to Pitta)
  Location: The point is located at a distance of 1 anguli proximal to TD 5
  between the radius and ulna.
  Indications: Constipation, sudden hoarseness, tinnitus, deafness, vomiting,
  pain and sensation of heaviness in shoulder and back.
  Puncture: The needle is inserted perpendicularly to 0.7 - 1 anguli depth.
  Can be treated with *agnikarma*.

* TD 7 (Cleft–*Antara* sira)

Location: The point is located at a distance of 3 angulis proximal to the wrist on the radial side of the ulna.

Indications: Epilepsy, deafness, pain of the upper limbs.

Puncture: The needle is inserted perpendicularly to ½ - 1 anguli depth. Can be treated with *agnikarma*.

* TD 8

Location: The point is located at a distance of 1 angulis proximal to TD 6, between the radius and ulna.

Indications: Deafness, sudden hoarseness, pain in the rib, hand and arm.

Puncture: The needle is inserted perpendicularly to ½ - 1 anguli depth. Can be treated with *agnikarma*.

* TD 9

Part of Indrabasti Marma (with P 6 and P 4). Sira of Jathara Agni and AnnaVaha Srotas.)

Location: The point is located between the radius and ulna at a distance of 5 angulis below the olecranon.

Indications: Deafness, underling hoarseness, pain in the hand and arm.

Puncture: The needle is inserted perpendicularly to ½ - 1 anguli depth. Can be treated with *agnikarma*.

* **TD 10 (Sea, *Samudra* sira, Earth *Prithvi* element point, sedation point. Sira related to Kapha along with the Sea (*Water*) sira of the Pericardium channel)**

Part of Kurpara Marma (with SI 8 and LI 11)

Location: The point is located in the depression 1 anguli above the olecranon (when elbow is flexed).

Indications: Epilepsy, unilateral headache, cardiac pain, cough, asthma, intercostal neuralgia, scrofula, upper quadrant pain, neck, shoulder and arm.

Kurpara Marma Therapy: Numbness of arm, pain in elbow, cardiac pain, cough, asthma.

Puncture: The needle is inserted perpendicularly to 0.3 - ½ anguli depth. Can be treated with *agnikarma*.

* TD 11

Part of Ani Marma (with LI 12 and L 4)

Location: The point is located at a distance of 2 angulis above the olecranon.

Indications: Pain and disorders in the shoulder and arm.

Ani Marma Therapy: Controls muscle tone.

Puncture: The needle is inserted perpendicularly to 0.3 anguli depth. Can be treated with *agnikarma*.

TD 12

Location: The point is located between TD 11 and TD 13.
Indications: Headache, stiffness and pain in the neck and arm.
Puncture: The needle is inserted perpendicularly to ½ -0.7 anguli depth. Can be treated with *agnikarma*.

TD 13

Location: The point is located at a distance of 3 angulis below TD 14.
Indications: Goiter, pain in the shoulder and arm.
Puncture: The needle is inserted perpendicularly to ½ -0.8 anguli depth. Can be treated with *agnikarma*.

* TD 14

Part of Kakshadhara Marma

Location: The point is located in depression, at a distance of 1 anguli posterior to LI 15 in the inferior-posterior part of the acromion.
Indications: Sensation of heaviness and immobility of shoulder, arm pain.
Kakshadhara Marma Therapy: It treats the muscle tone in the upper abdomen and chest.
Puncture: The needle is inserted perpendicularly or obliquely downward to 0.7 - 1 anguli depth. Can be treated with *agnikarma*.

TD 15

Location: The point is located midway between GB 21 and SI 13.
Indications: Rigidity and pain in neck, shoulder, arm.
Puncture: The needle is inserted perpendicularly to 0.3 - ½ anguli depth. Can be treated with *agnikarma*.

* TD 16

Part of Matrika Marma (with G 15, GB 21, LI 17 and C 23)

Location: The point is located level with SI 17 and UB 10, at the angle of the jaw.
Indications: Blurred vision, dizziness, facial edema, sudden deafness, neck stiffness.
Matrika Marma Therapy: Enhances circulation in the head. Controls *Majjavaha Srotas* (channels of the nervous system).
Puncture: The needle is inserted perpendicularly to 0.3 - ½ anguli depth. Can be treated with *agnikarma*.

* TD 17
Part of Vidhura Marma
   Location: The point is located in the depression, behind the earlobe.
   Indications: Disorders of the ears (tinnitus, deafness), edema of the cheeks, facial paralysis, lockjaw.
   Vidhura Marma Therapy: Ear diseases, facial paralysis.
   Puncture: The needle is inserted perpendicularly to ½ - 1 anguli depth. Can be treated with *agnikarma*.

TD 18
   Location: The point is located posterior to the helix of the ear, in the center of the mastoid process.
   Indications: Disorders of the ears (tinnitus, deafness), headache.
   Puncture: The needle is inserted obliquely to 0.1 anguli depth. Can be treated with *agnikarma*.

TD 19
   Location: The point is located behind the ear, around the level of the anti-helix.
   Indications: Disorders of the ears (tinnitus, ear pain), headache.
   Puncture: The needle is inserted obliquely to 0.1 anguli depth. Can be treated with *agnikarma*.

* TD 20
   Location: The point is located directly above the apex of the ear when it's bent, in the hairline.
   Indications: Endocrine disorders, edema, eye pain, dental pain, ear red and swollen ear, swollen and red eyes.
   Puncture: The needle is inserted obliquely to 0.1 anguli depth. Can be treated with *agnikarma*.

* TD 21
   Location: The point is located a distance of ½ anguli above the condyle of the jaw, in the anterior depression between the ear and the jaw joint.
   Indications: Ear disorders (deafness, tinnitus, ear), toothache.
   Puncture: The needle is inserted perpendicularly to 0.3 - ½ anguli depth. Can be treated with *agnikarma*.

TD 22
   Location: The point is located at a distance of 1 anguli in front of the root of the ear, in the anterior-superior part of the point TD 21.
   Indications: Sensation of heaviness of the head, headache, tinnitus, contraction of m. masseter.
   Puncture: The needle is inserted obliquely to 0.1-0.3 anguli depth avoiding the superficial temporal artery. Can be treated with *agnikarma*.

* TD 23

Part of Apanga Marma (with GB 1)
    Location: The point is located in the depression located at the outer end of the eyebrow.
    Indications: Disorders of eyes, (blurred vision, red and sore eyes), twitching of the eyelids, headache.
    Apanga Marma Therapy: Reduces nervous stress and can treat defective vision.
    Puncture: The needle is inserted horizontally towards the back to 0.3 anguli depth.

Nadis (*Extraordinary*)

CONCEPTION VESSEL (*Janma*) (Figures 27 and 30)

Channel Name: *Artava Nadi (or Janma Nadi)*
    Organ: Extraordinary organ of the reproductive system
    Related Nadi: *Sushumna*
    Channel location: Front of torso
    Siras number: 24
    Energy Flow: *Ascending*. Receives Prana from the Sushumna Nadi. Transmits Prana to the anterior part of the torso, it has an ascending flow and forms a circuit with the Shukra Nadi which has also an ascending flow but on the back of the torso. This flow is separated from the twelve channels- dhamanis.

Siras of Artava Nadi
Indications and location of the points of Artava Nadi:
    The Srotas also reflect their conditions in the Artava Nadi points besides the 12 organs. These Siras can treat problems in the srotas. * Demonstrates siras used often.

* C 1 (Part of Guda marma) Base Chakra (Muladhara) (with G 1)
    Location: The point is located in the space between the anus and the organs of generation. Center of the perineum. It's in the same area as the Earth *Chakra*.
    Indications: Mental disorders, pain and swelling of the anus, vulval itching, irregular menstruation, enuresis, spermatorrhea.
    Guda Marma Therapy: This is also the local *Apana Vayu sira* in the torso. Controls defecation and flatulence. It stimulates the uro-genital functions. Treats urinary and menstruation problems.
    Puncture: The needle is inserted perpendicularly to half anguli depth. Can be treated with *agnikarma*.

* C 2 (Sira which controls Apana Vayu, Medovaha Srotas and Shukravaha Srotas)

Location: The point is located in the front of the body directly above the symphysis pubis.

Indications: Impotence, leucorrhea, hernia and retention of urine.

Puncture: The needle is inserted perpendicularly a maximum of 1 anguli depth. Can be treated with *agnikarma*.

* C 3 (Front Urinary Bladder point and Mutravaha Srotas. Sira which controls Ambhuvaha Srotas)

Part of Basti Marma (Next to C 4, 5 and 6)

Location: The point is located in the front of the body 4 angulis directly below the navel.

Indications: Leucorrhea, irregular menstruation, hernia and retention of urine. Prolapse of the uterus.

Basti Marma Therapy: Diseases of the genito-urinary. Treatment of this *Marma* helps to stimulate *Kapha*.

Puncture: The needle is inserted perpendicularly, less than a maximum of 1 anguli depth. Can be treated with *agnikarma*.

* C 4 (Front point of the Small Intestine (Laghvantra) and Artavaha Srotas

Part of Basti Marma (with C 3, 5 and 6)

Location: The point is located at a distance of 3 angulis below the navel in the front of the body.

Indications: Leucorrhoea, dysmenorrhea, hernia and retention of urine.

Basti Marma Therapy: Diseases of the genito-urinary tract. Treatment of this *Marma* helps to stimulate *Kapha*.

Puncture: The needle is inserted perpendicularly to a maximum of 1 anguli depth. Can be treated with *agnikarma*.

* C 5 (Front point of the Tridosha (Sleshamashaya) and Shukravaha Srotas

Part of Basti Marma (with C 3, 4 and 6)

Location: The point is located at a distance of 2 angulis directly below the navel, on the front body.

Indications: Leucorrhoea, amenorrhea, hernia, edema and urine retention.

Basti Marma Therapy: Diseases of the genito-urinary tract. Treatment of this *Marma* helps to stimulate *Kapha*.

Puncture: The needle is inserted perpendicularly to a maximum of 1 anguli depth. Can be treated with *agnikarma*.

* C 6 Basti Marma (with C 3, 4 and 5) Sexual Chakra (*Svadhishthana*)
Location: The point is located at a distance of 1 ½ angulis below the navel on the front of the body.
Indications: Impotence, leucorrhoea, hernia, edema and retention of urine, *Ojas* deficiency, constipation and diarrhea.
Basti Marma Therapy: Diseases of the genitourinary tract. Treatment of this *Marma* helps to stimulate *Kapha*.
Puncture: The needle is inserted perpendicularly to a maximum of 1 anguli depth. Can be treated with *agnikarma*.

C 7
Location: The point is located at a distance of 1 anguli below the navel on the front of the body.
Indications: Leucorrhoea, hernia, edema and urine retention, constipation and diarrhea.
Puncture: The needle is inserted perpendicularly to a maximum of 1 anguli depth.

C 8 (Navel) Nabhi Marma, Navel Chakra (*Manipura*), sira which controls Pachaka Pitta)
Location: The point is located at the umbilicus/navel.
Indications: Prolapse of the rectum, diarrhea and abdominal pain and noise,
Puncture: Contraindicated for puncture but *Agnikarma* can be used.

* C 9
Location: The point is located 1 anguli directly above the umbilicus, in front of the body.
Indications: Edema and pain and noises in the abdomen, difficult urination, fluid build-up and moisture *Kapha type*.
Puncture: The needle is inserted perpendicularly to a maximum of 1 anguli depth. Can be treated with *agnikarma*.

C 10
Location: The point is located at a distance of 2 angulis superior to the umbilicus, in front of the body.
Indications: Vomiting, dysentery and abdominal pain and noises.
Puncture: The needle is inserted perpendicularly to a maximum of 1 anguli depth. Can be treated with *agnikarma*.

C 11

Location: The point is located at a distance of 3 angulis superior to the umbilicus, in front of the body.
Indications: Edema, anorexia and abdominal pain.
Puncture: The needle is inserted perpendicularly to a maximum of 1 anguli depth. Can be treated with *agnikarma*.

* C 12 (Front point of the Stomach (Amashaya) and Annavaha Srotas, sira which controls Kledaka Kapha)

Location: The point is located at a distance of 4 angulis superior to the umbilicus, in front of the body.
Indications: Vomiting, dysentery and abdominal enlargement, excess *Kapha*.
Puncture: The needle is inserted perpendicularly to a maximum of ½ anguli depth. Can be treated with *agnikarma*.

C 13

Location: The point is located at a distance of 5 angulis above the umbilicus in the front of the body.
Indications: Vomiting, seizures, diarrhea and abdominal bloating.
Puncture: The needle is inserted perpendicularly to a maximum of 1 anguli depth. Can be treated with *agnikarma*.

* C 14 (Front point of the Heart (Hridaya) and Pranavaha Srotas)

Location: The point is located at a distance of 6 angulis above the umbilicus, in the front of the body.
Indications: Mental problems such as epilepsy, vomiting, nausea, pain in the cardiac region.
Puncture: The needle is inserted perpendicularly to a maximum of 1 anguli depth. Can be treated with *agnikarma*.

C 15

Location: The point is located at a distance of 7 angulis above the umbilicus, in front of the body or directly below the xiphoid process of the sternum.
Indications: Mental disorders such as epilepsy, pain in the cardiac region.
Puncture: The needle is inserted obliquely downward surface to 0.4 anguli depth.

C 16

Location: The point is located at the level of the fifth intercostal space at the front of the body directly at the sternum.
Indications: Difficulty in swallowing.
Puncture: The needle is inserted horizontally and down to a maximum of ½ anguli depth. Can be treated with *agnikarma*.

C 17 Hridaya Marma (Front point of the Pericardium (Talahridaya), Rasavaha Srotas and Heart Chakra (*Anahata*). Sira which controls Vyana Vayu, Sadhaka Pitta, RaktaVaha Srotas and StanyaVaha Srotas)
   Location: The point is located at the level of the fourth intercostal space and the nipples on the front of the body directly at the sternum.
   Indications: Problems with lactation, asthma and chest pains. Controls Pranic centrifugal flow (*Vyana Vayu*), breast disease, hypogalactia, mastitis.
   Hridaya Marma Therapy: Enables balance in circulation and respiration. Balances *Sattva, Rajas* and *Tamas* being their seats. Affects *Sadhaka Pitta* by causing fantasy and reality to be indistinguishable when it is flawed. Treats the Pericardium organ.
   Puncture: The needle is inserted horizontally and down to a maximum of ½ anguli depth. Can be treated with *agnikarma*.

C 18
   Location: The point is located the level of the third intercostal space at the front of the body directly at the sternum.
   Indications: Chest pains, asthma and cough.
   Puncture: The needle is inserted horizontally and down to a maximum of ½ anguli depth. Can be treated with *agnikarma*.

C 19
   Location: The point is located the level of the second intercostal space at the front of the body directly at the sternum.
   Indications: Chest pains, asthma and cough.
   Puncture: The needle is inserted horizontally and down to a maximum of ½ anguli depth. Can be treated with *agnikarma*.

C 20
   Location: The point is located the level of the first intercostal space at the front of the body directly at the sternum.
   Indications: Chest pains, asthma and cough.
   Puncture: The needle is inserted horizontally to a maximum of ½ anguli depth. Can be treated with *agnikarma*.

C 21
   Location: The point is located in the front of the body directly at the breastbone between the C 21 and the end of the sternum.
   Indications: Chest pains, asthma and cough.
   Puncture: The needle is inserted horizontally to a maximum of ½ anguli depth. Can be treated with *agnikarma*.

* C 22

Location: The point is located in the front of the body directly above the sternum, in the center of the suprasternal pit.

Indications: Sore throats, asthma and cough. It balances the sense of time and treats hoarseness and loss of taste.

Puncture: The needle is inserted horizontally to a maximum of ½ anguli depth. Can be treated with *agnikarma*.

* C 23 Nila Marma, Laryngeal Chakra (*Vishuddha*)

Location: The point is located in front of the body in the depression directly above the Adam's apple.

Indications: Problems with the tongue, difficulty in swallowing and loss of voice.

Nila Marma Therapy: Balances sense of time and treats hoarseness and loss of taste. Controls *Majjavaha Srotas* (channels of the nervous system).

Puncture: The needle is inserted perpendicularly and upward to 1 anguli depth.

* C 24

Location: The point is located in front of the body in the depression directly in the center between the lower lip and chin.

Indications: Problems with tongue, difficulty in swallowing and loss of voice, mental disorders, stiff neck.

Puncture: The needle is inserted perpendicularly and upward, maximum of 1 anguli depth. Can be treated with *agnikarma*.

GOVERNOR or MINISTER
(*Amatya*) NADI (Figures 26 and 27)

Channel Name: *Shukra Nadi (or Amatya Nadi)*

Organ: Extraordinary organ of the mental and nerve systems

Related Nadi: *Sushumna*

Channel location: Back of torso

Siras number: 28

Energy Flow: *Ascending*. Receives Prana from Sushumna Nadi. Transmits Prana to the back of the torso and head, has ascending flow and forms a circuit with the Artava Nadi flow which also has influence but in this case on the anterior part of the torso. This flow is separate from the twelve channels, the dhamanis' flow.

Shukra Nadi Siras

Indications and location of the points of Shukra nadi (G): * *Demonstrates siras used often.*

* G 1 (Part of Guda marma) Base Chakra (*Muladhara*)

Location: The point is located between the tip of the coccyx and the anus. It relates to the first *chakra*.

Indications: Constipation, diarrhea, hemorrhoids, sore lower back and prolapse of the rectum.

Guda Marma Therapy: This is also the local *Apana Vayu* sira on the torso. Controls defecation and flatulence. It stimulates the uro-genital functions.

Puncture: The needle is inserted perpendicularly no more than one anguli depth. Can be treated with *agnikarma*.

* G 2 (Part of Guda marma) Base Chakra (*Muladhara*)

Location: The point is located in the hollow of the sacrum.

Indications: Pain and restriction of movement of the lower back, hemorrhoids, epilepsy.

Guda Marma Therapy: This is also the local *Apana Vayu* sira on the torso. Controls defecation and flatulence. It stimulates the uro-genital functions.

Puncture: The needle is inserted obliquely and superficially to ½ anguli depth. Can be treated with *agnikarma*.

* G 3 (Sexual Chakra (*Svadhishthana*) posterior point)

Location: The point is located at the end point of the spiny apophysis of the fourth lumbar vertebra.

Indications: Seminal emission, irregular menstruation, impotence and pain and restriction of movement of the lower back.

Puncture: The needle is inserted perpendicularly to a maximum of 1 anguli depth. Can be treated with *agnikarma*.

* G 4

Location: The point is located at the end point of the spiny apophysis of the second lumbar vertebra.

Indications: Diarrhea, seminal emission, impotence, stiff back, female disorders (prolapse of the uterus, leucorrhoea).

Puncture: The needle is inserted perpendicularly to a maximum of 1 anguli depth. Can be treated with *agnikarma*.

G 5

Location: The point is located at the end point of the spiny apophysis of the first lumbar vertebra.

Indications: Epilepsy, restriction of movement and back pain, diarrhea.

Puncture: The needle is inserted perpendicularly to a maximum of 1 anguli depth. Can be treated with *agnikarma*.

* **G 6 (Navel Chakra (*Manipura*) posterior point)**
  Location: The point is located at the end point of the spiny apophysis of the eleventh thoracic vertebra.
  Indications: Hemorrhoids, epilepsy. It can be used to relax muscles in the area.
  Puncture: The needle is inserted perpendicularly to a maximum of 1 anguli depth.

G 7
  Location: The point is located at the end point of the spiny apophysis of the tenth thoracic vertebra.
  Indications: Restriction of movement and back pain.
  Puncture: The needle is inserted perpendicularly to a maximum of 1 anguli depth. Can be treated with *agnikarma*.

G 8
  Location: The point is located at the end point of the spiny apophysis of the ninth thoracic vertebra.
  Indications: Restriction of motion of the back, abdominal pain, epilepsy.
  Puncture: The needle is inserted perpendicularly to a maximum of 1 anguli depth. Can be treated with *agnikarma*.

G 9
  Location: The point is located at the end point of the spiny apophysis of the seventh thoracic vertebra.
  Indications: Restriction of movement and back pain. Asthma and cough.
  Puncture: The needle is inserted obliquely upwards and superficially to maximum of 1 anguli depth. Can be treated with *agnikarma*.

* **G 10 (Heart Chakra (*Anahata*), posterior point)**
  Location: The point is located at the end point of the spiny apophysis of the sixth thoracic vertebra.
  Indications: Restriction of movement in back and neck pain, asthma and cough.
  Puncture: The needle is inserted perpendicularly to a maximum of 1 anguli depth. Can be treated with *agnikarma*.

* **G 11**
  Location: The point is located at the end point of the spiny apophysis of the fifth thoracic vertebra.
  Indications: Cough, restriction of movement and back pain, anxiety and lack of memory.
  Puncture: The needle is inserted perpendicularly to a maximum of 1 anguli depth. Can be treated with *agnikarma*.

G 12

    Location: The point is located at the end point of the spiny apophysis of the third thoracic vertebra.

    Indications: Restriction of movement and back pain, asthma, cough and epilepsy.

    Puncture: The needle is inserted perpendicularly to a maximum of 1 anguli depth. Can be treated with *agnikarma*.

G 13

    Location: The point is located at the end point of the spiny apophysis of the first thoracic vertebra.

    Indications: Fever, headaches and neck pain.

    Puncture: The needle is inserted perpendicularly to a maximum of 1 anguli depth. Can be treated with *agnikarma*.

* G 14 (Laryngeal Chakra (*Vishuddha*), posterior point (Sira that controls Asthi Dhatu and Ojas)

    Location: The point is located between the endpoint of the spiny apophysis of the first thoracic vertebra and the seventh cervical vertebra.

    Indications: Cough, sore throat, asthma, colds, febrile diseases and immunity, epilepsy. It influences *Asthi Dhatu*.

    Puncture: The needle is inserted perpendicularly to a maximum of 1 anguli depth. Can be treated with *agnikarma*.

G 15 (Controls Purishavaha Srotas)
Part of Matrika Marma (next to TD 16, GB 20, SI 17 and C 23).

    Location: The point is located in the depression below the border of the edge of the skull near the G 16 which is ½ anguli above G 15. Dangerous point.

    Indications: Mental problems, aphonia, aphasia. Loss of neck movement and functions in the area of the head which can result in unconsciousness.

    Matrika Marma Therapy: Enhances circulation in the head. Controls *Majjavaha Srotas* (channels of the nervous system).

    Puncture: The needle is inserted perpendicularly to a maximum of 1 anguli depth. Deep insertion is contraindicated.

* G 16 (Krikatika marma, posterior point of Ajna Chakra)

    Location: The point is located in the lower depression at the border of the edge of the skull over half anguli G 15. Dangerous point.

    Indications: Mental problems, aphonia, aphasia. Loss of neck movement and functions in the area of the head which can result in unconsciousness.

    Krikatika Marma Therapy: Neck and shoulder pain, mental problems.

    Puncture: The needle is inserted perpendicularly to a maximum of 1 anguli depth. Deep insertion is contraindicated.

G 17

Location: The point is located at a distance of a 1 ½ anguli above the edge of the skull.
Indications: Dizziness, restriction of movement and neck pain, epilepsy.
Puncture: The needle is inserted horizontally with the skin, up to ½ anguli depth. Can be treated with *agnikarma*.

G 18

Location: The point is located at a distance of 1 ½ anguli above G 17.
Indications: Restriction of movement of neck, headache, vision problems, epilepsy.
Puncture: The needle is inserted horizontally with the skin, up to ½ anguli depth. Can be treated with *agnikarma*.

G 19

Location: The point is located at a distance of 1 ½ anguli above G 18.
Indications: Dizziness, headache.
Puncture: The needle is inserted horizontally with the skin, up to ½ anguli depth. Can be treated with *agnikarma*.

* G 20 (Adhipati marma, Crown Chakra (*Sahasrara*) (meeting point of all dhamanis)

Location: The point is located at a distance of 1 ½ anguli above G 19. Point is at the junction which is formed from a line directed from the lobe to the apex of the two ears until the two lines intersect at the middle of the skull.
Indications: Headaches, ringing in the ears. *Prana Vata disorders.*
Adhipati Marma Therapy: Treatment of psychiatric diseases and diseases of the nervous system, balances *prana*, the pineal gland and is useful in diseases of the nervous system. Headaches, ringing in the ears.
Puncture: The needle is inserted obliquely or horizontally to a maximum of ½ anguli depth. Can be treated with *agnikarma*.

G 21

Location: The point is located at a distance of 1 ½ anguli anterior to G 20.
Indications: Blurred vision, dizziness and headaches.
Puncture: The needle is inserted horizontally to a maximum of ½ anguli depth. Can be treated with *agnikarma*.

* G 22 (Part of Shringataka marma (with G 23)

Location: The point is located at a distance of 3 angulis anterior to G 20.
Indications: Treats the nervous system and soothes the eyes, ears, nose and tongue.
Shringataka Marma Therapy: Stimulates the nervous system and balances the eyes, ears, nose and tongue.
Puncture: The needle is inserted horizontally to a maximum of ½ anguli depth. Can be treated with *agnikarma*.

* **G 23 (Part of Shringataka marma (with G 22)**
  Location: The point is located at a distance of 1 anguli anterior to G 22.
  Indications: Treats the nervous system and soothes the eyes, ears, nose and tongue.
  Shringataka Marma Therapy: Stimulates the nervous system and balances the eyes, ears, nose and tongue.
  Puncture: The needle is inserted horizontally to a maximum of ½ anguli depth. Can be treated with *agnikarma*.

G 24
  Location: The point is located at a distance of 1 anguli anterior to G 23.
  Indications: Pain, headache, vertigo, insomnia, anxiety, heart palpitations.
  Puncture: The needle is inserted horizontally and upwardly to a maximum of ½ anguli depth. Can be treated with *agnikarma*.

* **G 24.5 (Sthapani Marma, Brow Chakra (*Ajna*). Sira which controls Pranavaha Srotas)**
  Location: The point is located between the two eyebrows.
  Indications: Relates with the pituitary gland and a primary site of Prana. Location of the Brow *Chakra*.
  Puncture: The needle is inserted obliquely and superficially downwards to 0.4 anguli depth.

* **G 25 (Sira which controls Majjavaha Srotas)**
  Location: The point is located at the end of the nose.
  Indications: Nasal obstruction and epistaxis.
  Puncture: The needle is inserted perpendicularly to a maximum of 0.3 anguli depth.

* **G 26**
  Location: The point is located below the nose, in the depression above the upper lip.
  Indications: For acute emergencies, seizures, fainting, epilepsy, shock.
  Puncture: The needle is inserted obliquely up to a maximum of 0.3 anguli depth.

G 27 (Sira which controls Majjavaha Srotas)
  Location: The point is located on the edge of the upper lip.
  Indications: Sore gums and lips.
  Puncture: The needle is inserted perpendicularly to a maximum of 0.3 anguli depth.

* **G 28**

Location: The point is located between the gum and lip.

Indications: Pain and swelling of gums.

Puncture: The needle is inserted obliquely and upward to a maximum of 0.3 anguli depth.

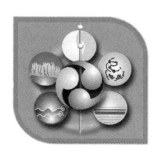

AYURVEDA & ACUPUNCTURE

Conclusion

Ayurvedic acupuncture is almost a lost art. This has been caused by many factors including wars, invasions and colonialism of India. The only surgical techniques (of which acupuncture can be considered a therapy) allowed for a long time was the allopathic method, so it's fair to conclude that needles and needle piercing were also banned.

Efforts over the last few years to revive it have been positive but like anything worthwhile in life, it takes time. Often it has to overcome the prejudices of those who do not understand it but this is a normal thing in Science. Most positive discoveries in Science have almost never been readily accepted by the establishment until many years later.

Ayurvedic acupuncture can add a further dimension in clinical practice, especially for those who utilize Ayurveda. Understanding an acupuncture system which has the same terminologies and principles is always easier and more holistic in practice than constantly using foreign systems which although may share many common points, can also be confusing.

Marmapuncture, the common name for Ayurvedic acupuncture does not only deal with treatment of physical diseases or organs but can also balance emotions and psychological imbalances. Consequently, it is a whole body therapy which can treat the seven bodies or koshas of Ayurveda.

It is rewarding to see that great interest in marmapuncture is occurring in the West. This seems to be a natural process in that for most systems to be totally accepted in their own home country, they need to be firstly promoted in the West, especially the USA. Ayurveda is not different, since the great interest in India has been strengthened and fueled for the most part by Western interest in the subject. This originally occurred with Yoga, which was not until the German psychologists became interested in the subject, that the world followed. This also applies to Kalaripayyat, the ancient Indian martial art, which was almost hardly known in India but today is experiencing a great revival, which occurred after a BBC documentary on Kalaripayyat aired internationally.

In my first book, *The Lost Secrets of Ayurvedic Acupuncture*, I mentioned that it *"should stimulate further research and interest in an important [though neglected] branch of possibly the most ancient and comprehensive medical system in the world. It requires much effort on the part of other Ayurvedic researchers to enhance and expand it so as to create a source of continuity for the present and future health of the human race."* (Ros, p.161).

It is rewarding to see that this wish is coming to fruition by the important work of other Ayurvedic experts and researchers, including Joshi and Shah.

Frank J. Ros
Australia

About the Author

Dr. Frank Ros is a Doctor of Ayurvedic Medicine (Ayurveda Parangata) and is a qualified Naturopath, a professional member of the Complementary Medicine Association and of the Naturopathic Practitioners Association, also a founding member of the International Association of Ayurvedic Acupuncture. His first work on marmapuncture, a discipline in which he's a specialist was published in the United Sates of America in 1994; *The Lost Secrets of Ayurvedic Acupuncture* published by Lotus Press and by several other foreign language publishers. In 2008 he published Marmapuntura in Argentina, for the first time in Spanish. Dr. Ros resides in Australia and regularly visits the US and Argentina to give lectures and seminars.

He can be contacted at webmarma@internode.on.net or via the website: www.marmapuncture.com.au

Using Marmapuncture in practice

New York

Dr. Frank Ros has been my principal instructor in Ayurvedic acupuncture in the United States for ten years. I'm a naturopathic doctor and licensed acupuncturist in three states of the US and certified by the National Commission of Acupuncture and Oriental Medicine and I find that Frank's knowledge of acupuncture and the ability to teach it is second to none. He is the leading exponent of Ayurvedic acupuncture in the world and his written works and his lectures set the standard for this important part of Ayurvedic medicine and integrative care. He has been the advisor for our Ayurvedic acupuncture program and Ayurvedic medicine program at Clifton Springs Hospital in Clifton Springs, NY, for a number of years. We have used him as a clinical and an academic advisor for our clinical and residential programs.

Dr. Les Moore
ND, MSOM, LAc.
Director, Integrative Medicine
Clifton Springs Hospital and Clinic
Clifton Springs, NY 14432

Australia

I have an advanced diploma of Ayurveda from The Australian Institute of Holistic Medicine, a nationally registered and accredited college in Australia. My clinical studies also took me to the Dharmasthala SDM Ayurveda Hospital in Udupi Kanataka, India where I performed intensive clinical practice for a period of two months, an invaluable experience.

As a practitioner of Ayurveda I find it most beneficial to have also completed the post graduate studies with Dr Frank Ros in Marma Therapy/Marmapuncture.

I have since been using the ancient teachings of marmapuncture (siravedhana) with great success, in a wide variety of cases.

The marmapuncture course did tie in very well with my previous knowledge of Ayurveda. It was easy to understand and apply to the general Ayurvedic understanding of the body systems with the doshas and their subtypes, as well as dhatus and srotas.

I personally find that the marmapuncture course taught by Dr. Ros has given me a great advantage in not only the fact that I have a very powerful extra therapy that I can use on my clients, but it has also enhanced my sensitivity and understanding of marmas and the channels running through the body while I also do Ayurvedic massage. I have clients who comment that they feel a deep healing happening during the treatment and that when I work on certain marmapoints they feel deeply nourished by the touch in places where they always have wanted to be touched.

My experience with the outcome of using marmapuncture on my clients has by far exceeded any expectations I might have previously had. As I use marmapuncture in combination with herbal treatment and life style advice, I can truly say that I have been extremely surprised and excited about how quickly I have seen my clients improve to the point where in a short time, they do not need to come for treatments any longer.

I am currently treating a client with hyperhidrosis who notices a distinct difference in her state of being if she does not come for marmapuncture on a weekly basis, for the moment. This particular client first came to me for some suspected infertility problems although she is only 27 years of age. She had only had very scanty and irregular periods for 1 year since coming off the pill. After treating her with herbs and marmapuncture, she was menstruating after just 3 weeks and is now following a regular cycle of 28 days, menstruating at the correct moon phase starting just before the New moon.

Another of my clients that I treated with marmapuncture over a period of 4 weeks about 3 months ago, claims that the treatment has improved her general health and the specific complaints that she came for so much so, that she feels the treatments have literally changed her life. She is now keen to learn Ayurveda and Marmapuncture herself. She suffered from anxiety, liver problems, high cholesterol, was overweight with difficulty loosing weight and lack of energy, especially in the afternoon. She now feels no anxiety, has more energy than she has experienced for years, she has lost weight, is motivated to exercise and generally feels really well.

Yet another client I treated with marmapuncture became so well in a record space of time that she went on to win the Australian national championship in figure skating a week after her last treatment. She had for 3 years been suffering from extreme motion sickness. Every plane trip, car ride even being in a pool or getting up too early in the morning would make her feel dizzy, nauseated and often would make her throw up and be bedridden for at least 24 hours, often longer. I gave her general anti Vata treatment with herbs and lifestyle advice for 5 weeks. She had only 2 marmapuncture treatments, the last one less than a week before her competition. She experienced no motion sickness or dizziness following her flight to compete in Melbourne. She on the other hand felt very fit and strong and focused, and did go on to win the competition for the first time in 16 years of competing in the sport.

I have myself experienced very good results from exchanging marmapuncture with my fellow students and now colleagues. My lower back pain and tension has been reduced by 80-90%, and my knees that have been painful for a while since a skiing injury a few years back, have improved.

Karina Thullesen
Advanced Diploma of Ayurveda. Postgrad Ayur.Acupuncture
Fremantle, Western Australia
18 March, 2013

Bibliography

Bishagratna, K.L. *Sushruta Samhita*, Chowkhambha Sanskrit Series Office, Varanasi, India. 1991.

Dash, B. *Ayurveda For Mother and Child*. Delhi Diary Pub., India. 1988.

Feuerstein, G. *The Textbook of Yoga*. Rider and Co., London. 1975.

Frawley, D. *Ayurvedic Healing*. Passage Press, Utah USA, 1989.

Frawley, D. *Ayurveda and the Mind*. Lotus Press. NM USA, 1997.

Frawley, D. Ranade, S. Lele, A. *Ayurveda and Marma Therapy*. Lotus Press. Wi, USA. 2003.

Frawley, D. Ranade, S. Lele, A. *Secrets of Marma*. Inter. Acad. Ayur, Poona, India, 1999.

Godagama, S. *The Handbook of Ayurveda*. Kyle Cathie Ltd. London. 2001.

Iyengar, B.K.S. *Light on Pranayama*. Unwin Paperbacks London.1981.

Jayasuriya, A. *Clinical Acupuncture*. B. Jain Publishers, India 7th edition 1994.

Jayasuriya, A. *Clinical Acupuncture*. Medicina Alternativa International, Sri Lanka. 15th Edition.

Joshi, B. Shah, R. and Joshi, G. *Vedic Health Care System* (Clinical Practice of Sushrutokta Marma Chikitsa and Siravedhana-highlighting Acupuncture). New Age Books, New Delhi. Including FOREWORD by Dr. H.S. Sharma. 2002.

Kulkarni, P.H. *Probable Links Between Ayurveda and Acupuncture*. I.I.M. Pune. India. 1985.

Lad, V. *Ayurveda, The Science of Self-Healing*. Lotus Press. Wi USA 1985.

Lad, V. and Frawley, D. *Yoga of Herbs*, Lotus Press. Wi. USA. 1986.

Nagpal C.L. *Modern Acupuncture*, Acupuncture Society of India Publishing, Jaipur, India. 1984.

Omura, Yoshiaki. *Acupuncture Medicine*. Japan Publications Inc. Tokyo, Japan. 1982.

Ranade, S. Lele, A. Frawley, D. *Secrets of Marma*. International Academy of Ayurveda Publishing, Pune India. 1999.

Ranade, S. *Natural Healing Through Ayurveda*, Passage Press, Utah USA. 1993.

Reid, H. and Croucher M. *The Way Of the Warrior*. Century Publishing, London. 1986.

Ros, Frank. *The Lost Secrets of Ayurvedic Acupuncture*, Lotus Press, U.S.A. 1994.

Sharma R.K. and Dash B. *Charaka Samhita*, Chaukhamba Orientalia, India 1976.

Shealy, Norman. *The Complete Illustrated Encyclopedia of Alternative Healing Therapies*. C. Element Publishing, Boston. USA 1999.

Svoboda, R. *Ayurveda, Life, Health and Longevity*. Arkana Publishers USA 1992.

Svoboda, R. *Prakruti, Your Ayurvedic Constitution*. Geocom Pub. N.M. USA.1999.

Svoboda, R. Lade, A. *Tao and Dharma*. Lotus Press, Wi USA.1995.

Thatte, D.G. *Acupuncture Marma and Other Asian Therapeutic Techniques*. Chaukhambha Orientalia, Delhi. 1988.

Tiwari, M. *Ayurveda Secrets of Healing*. Lotus Press. Twin Lakes USA 1995.

Veltheim, John. *Acupuncture*. Hill of Content Publishing. Melb. Australia 1985.

Wexu, M. *A Modern Guide to Ear Acupuncture*. Appendix by Dr. C. Thakkur, Aurora Press N.M. USA 1985.

Glossary

ACUPUNCTURE
The system of puncturing the pressure points for therapy.

ADANKAL
Pressure points and its therapies, especially in Kerala (India).

AGNI
Digestive fire.

AGNI KARMA
Heat therapy, moxibustion.

AHAMKARA
Ego.

AJNA CHAKRA
Energy vortex between eyebrows.

AKASHA
Ether, space, material, one of the Five Elements.

ALAMBA CHAKRA
Wheel of Support of the 5 Elements.

ALOCHAKA PITTA
Pitta in the eyes governing vision.

AMA
Undigested food particles transformed into toxins.

AMASHAYA
Stomach.

ANAHATA CHAKRA
Energy vortex centering in the heart region.

ANTAR NADIS
Solid organ related channels.

AP
Another name for the Water element.

APANA VAYU
Energy relating to downward movement in the body.

ASHAYA DHAMANIS
Channels with an ascending flow of energy.

ASHTANGA AYURVEDA
The Ayurvedic 8 classical specialties

ASHTANGA HRIDAYA
Ancient text attributed to Vagbhatta.

ASTHI
Bone, one of the seven tissues.

ATHARVA VEDA
One of the 4 Vedas

AVLAMBAKA KAPHA
Kapha in the lung and heart which lubricates the thorax.

AYURVEDA
The Science of Life. Traditional medicine of India.

AYUS
Life.

BAHU
Arms.

BAHYA NADIS
Channels directly related to the hollow organs.

BHEDANA KARMA
Therapy via puncturing.

BHUTA AGNI
The 5 biological fires in the liver.

BODHAKA KAPHA
Kapha in the mouth which controls taste.

BHRAJAKA PITTA
Pitta on the skin.

BUDDHISM
Indian religious philosophy.

CHAKRA
Centers or vortices of energy, also a wheel and a cycle.

CHARAKA
Ancient Ayurvedic doctor, author of the *Samhita* named after him.

CHI
The life force in Chinese medicine equivalent to Ayurvedic prana.

DARSHANA
Observation, part of Ayurvedic diagnosis.

DHANUR VEDA
The Science of War. Ancient Indian text of the martial arts.

DHAMANI
Channel or meridian through which Prana o Rasa flows to the *siras* or acupuncture points.

DHATUS
Tissues, the 7 Tissues.

DHATU CHAKRA
Wheel of the tissues, its circuit.

DHATU DHAMANIS
Channels or meridians which have an ascending flow of prana.

DOSHA
Biological force(s), humor(s) responsible for health and disease.

GRAHANI
Small Intestine.

GUNAS
Attributes, characteristics.

GUNA DVANDVA
The two opposing forces (like *yin* and *yang*).

HRIDAYA
The heart.

IDA
Energetic channel that behaves like Kapha and affects the left side of the body.

JALA
The element of Water.

JANMA
Meridian or nadi of conception also named Artava Nadi.

JIHVA
Tongue diagnosis.

KALARI
Ancient Indian martial art. Also *kalaripayyat*.

KAPHA
Biological humor relating to the elements of Water and Earth, phlegm.

KARNA
The ear, ear diagnosis.

KASH
To radiate, part of the word Akasha (ether).

KLEDAKA KAPHA
Kapha in the stomach which looks after the first stage of digestion.

KOSTHANGAS
The physical organs especially in the torso.

KURCCHA
Marma in the foot and hand.

MAJJA
Nerve tissue and medulla.

MAMSA
Muscle, one of the 7 tissues.

MANIPURA CHAKRA
Energy vortex in the navel.

MARMA
107 vital points. Large centers or zones of accumulation of prana as well as being vital or sensitive zones to trauma and injury. Each marma has one or more siras.

MARMA ADI
Martial art system specializing in strikes to the vital points.

MARMA CHIKITSA
Treatment or therapy of the marmas or vital points.

MARMAPUNCTURE
Acupuncture of the Marmas.

MEDA
Fat, one of the 7 tissues.

MOXIBUSTION
Heat therapy.

MULADHARA CHAKRA
Energy vortex at the base of the spinal column.

MULA SIRAS
Base vital points where the energy is retained in the channel.

MUTRASHAYA
Urinary Bladder.

NADI
A channel or meridian that allows the transportation of prana to the 107 marma and chakras as well as to the sense organs.

NADI PARIKSHA
Pulse diagnosis.

NAGADAMANI
Artemisa Vulgaris

NALANDA
Ancient Indian University.

NEEDLING
Acupuncture.

NIRAMA
Without toxins.

NIRMANA CHAKRA
Wheel of Creation of the 5 Elements.

OJAS
Immunity, immune essence in the body.

PACHACA PITTA
Pitta that supports the other four Pittas.

PADA
Foot or leg.

PANCHA BHAUTIKA SIRAS
The acupoints of the Five Elements in each meridian/dhamani.

PANCHA KARMA
The five therapies of detoxification.

PANCHA MAHABHUTAS
The Five Great Elements. *Godai* in Japanese.

PANCHA SRU SIRAS
The acupoints of the Five Elements in each meridian/dhamani.

PHUPHUSA/FUFUSA
The lung.

PINGALA
Pitta related channel controlling the right side of the body.

PITAR/BALA
Parent-child concept of the Five Element points.

PITTA
Metabolic humor, bile.

PITTASHAYA
Gall bladder.

PLIHA
Spleen.

PRAKOPA
Aggravation of a humor.

PRAKRUTI
Constitution (Vata, Pitta, Kapha), the primordial matter.

PRANA
Life or vital energy.

PRANAYAMA
Breathing system of Yoga or Ayurveda.

PRANIC MANDALA
Ayurvedic biorhythmic clock.

PRASHAMA
Alleviation of a humor.

PRASHNA
Diagnosis questionnaire.

PRITHVI
The element of Earth.

PURUSHA
The primordial consciousness.

RAKTA
Blood.

RANJAKA PITTA
Pitta reddish secretions.

RAJAS
One of the mental humors, agitation.

RASA
Plasma, and also the name of prana, vital energy that circulates though the channels or meridians.

RIG VEDA
One of the 4 Vedas

SADHAKA PITTA
One of the Pittas that governs intelligence.

SAHASRA CHAKRA
Energy vortex on the crown of the head.

SAMA
State associated with ama or toxins.

SAMA VEDA
One of the 4 Vedas

SAMANA VAYU
Energy that affects the digestion.

SAMCHAYA
Accumulation of a humor.

SAMHITA
Classical Ayurvedic text.

SATTVA
Purity, one of the mental humors.

SETU SIRAS
Vital acupoints that form bridges between two related channels or dhamanis.

SHLESHMASHAYA
The Tridosha channel (3D).

SHALYA CHIKITSA
see *Shalya Tantra*

SHALYA TANTRA
Ayurvedic surgery.

SHASTRA
Text book.

SHUKRA
Semen, reproductive fluid.

SHRINGATIKA
One of the marmas.

SIRA
Point on the surface of the skin that communicates with the underlying meridian or channel (dhamani). Blood vessels.

SIRA-MATRIKA
Marma on the neck.

SIRAVEDHANA
Ayurvedic acupuncture. Term utilized by Sushruta.

SLESHAKA KAPHA
Kapha in the synovial fluid.

SPARSHANA
Palpation (in diagnosis).

SROTAS
Plural of Srotas.

Srotas
Subtle or gross channel that allows the flow of substances such as blood, energy etc.

STHAPANI
Brow Marma.

SUCHI
Acupuncture needle. *Suchika*-acupuncturist.

SUCHI CHIKITSA
Defining name of acupuncture in Ayurveda.

SUCHI VEDA
Science of acupuncture, ancient Indian acupuncture text book.

SUSHUMNA
Energy channel along the center of the spinal column.

SURYA
The Sun, a point in ear acupuncture that treats migraines.

SUSHRUTA
Ancient Ayurvedic surgeon and author of one of the *Samhitas*.

SVADISTHANA CHAKRA
Energy vortex centering the sexual organs.

TAKSHASHILA
Ancient Ayurvedic university.

TALAHRIDAYA
Pericardium and a marma.

TAMAS
One of the mental humors, inertia.

TANMATRAS
The smallest part of energy.

TARPAKA KAPHA
Kapha in the brain and heart.

TEJAS
The Fire element.

TIRYAG DHAMANIS
Channels or dhamanis which have a transversal flow of energy.

TRIDOSHA
The Science of the Three Humors, the three humors, the channel (dhamani) of the three humors, the three doshic zones in the torso.

UDANA VATA
Vata energy that supports expression and memory.

UPA VEDA
Subsidiary text of the Vedas.

VAGBHATTA
Great doctor and seer of Ayurveda in antiquity.

VATA
The catabolic humor, related to wind or air.

VAYU
Wind, motivator of energy, sometimes it refers to Vata.

VEDAS
Ancient sacred writings of India.

VINASHA CHAKRA
Wheel of Destruction of the Five Elements.

VINAYA CHAKRA
Wheel of Control of the Five Elements.

VISSUDHA CHAKRA
Energy vortex in the throat area.

VRIHDANTRA
Large Intestine.

VRIKKA
The kidney.

VYANA VAYU
The energy (Vata) that governs muscle movement, in the joints and circulation.

VYADHANA
Another name for Ayurvedic acupuncture. (Not commonly used).

YAJUR VEDA
One of the 4 Vedas.

YAKRT
The liver.

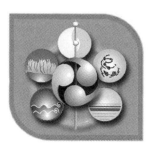

Index

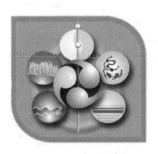

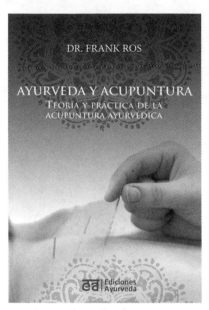

Ayurveda and Acupuncture
is also available in Spanish from
Ediciones Ayurveda, Barcelona, Spain.
contact@edicionesayurveda.com
www.edicionesayurveda.com

 The **International Academy of Ayurvedic Acupuncture** is a place of study or training in Ayurvedic Acupuncture. It is also an institution or society of distinguished scholars, practitioners and students that aim at promoting and maintaining acceptable standards in the practice of Ayurvedic Acupuncture, specifically and Ayurveda in general.

For further information:

email: iaayac@marmapuncture.com.au

website: www.marmapuncture.com.au

Lost Secrets of
Ayurvedic Acupuncture

by Dr. Frank Ros
ISBN: 9780914955122
206 pp pb • $15.95 Item# 990375

Ayurvedic Acupuncture is based upon the Suchi Veda, a 3,000 year old Vedic text which, in the Ayurvedic system, is the Science of Acupuncture. It has been practiced as an accessory therapy since it was used in conjunction with other forms to effect healing. It belongs more correctly to the branch of surgery, one of the eight medical discplines of Ayurveda.

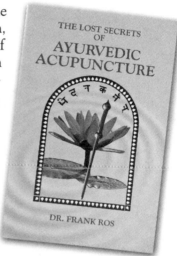

Available at bookstores and natural food stores nationwide or order your copy directly by sending cost of item plus $2.50 shipping/handling ($.75 s/h for each additional copy ordered at the same time) to:

Lotus Press, PO Box 325, Twin Lakes, WI 53181 USA
toll free order line: 800 824 6396 • office phone: 262 889 856 • office fax: 262 889 2461
email: lotuspress@lotuspress.com • web site: www.LotusPress.com

Lotus Press is the publisher of a wide range of books and software in the field of alternative health, including Ayurveda, Chinese medicine, herbology, aromatherapy, Reiki and energetic healing modalities. Request our free book catalog.